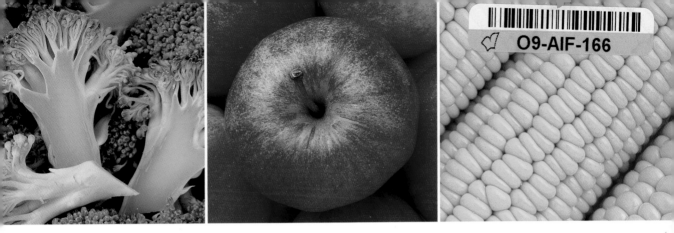

# THE**FOOD**DOCTOR

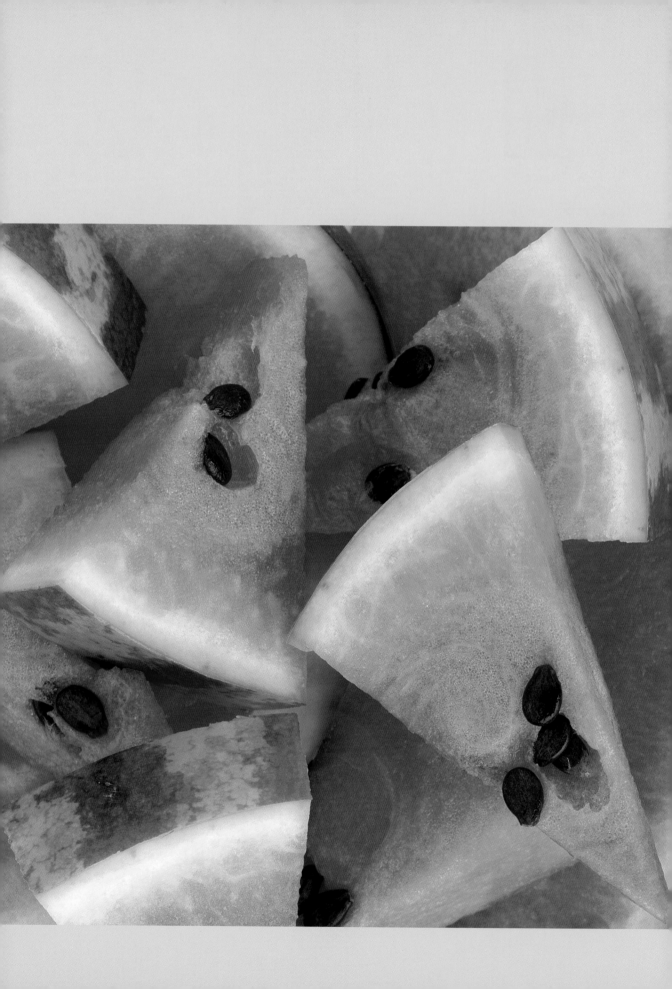

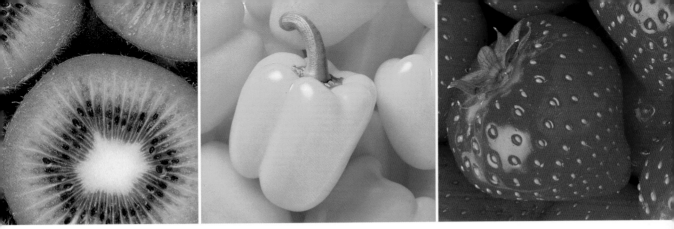

# THE**FOOD**DOCTOR

## Healing foods for mind and body

**Ian Marber** Dip ION **& Vicki Edgson** Dip ION

**Additional text by**
**Susan Perry** B.SC. HONS Dip ION

for more information
from The Food Doctor visit
**www.thefooddoctor.com**

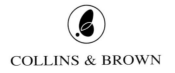

COLLINS & BROWN

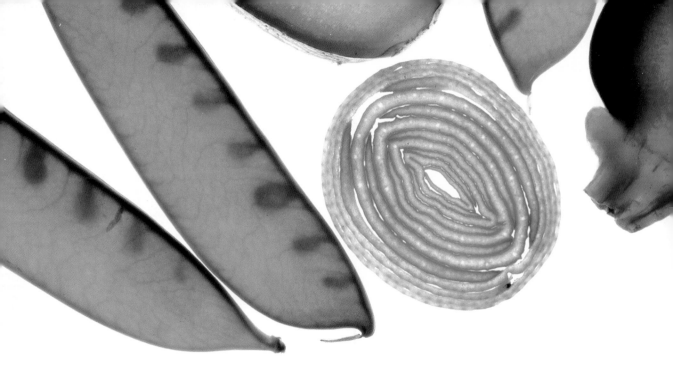

First published in Great Britain in 1999
Revised edition published in Great Britain in 2004
by Collins & Brown Ltd
The Chrysalis Building,
Bramley Road, London W10 6SP

An imprint of **Chrysalis** Books Group plc

Distributed in the United States and Canada by
Sterling Publishing Co., 387 Park Avenue South,
New York, NY 10016 USA

10 9 8 7 6 5 4 3 2 1

British Library Cataloguing-in-Publication Data:
A catalogue record for this book is available from the
British Library.

ISBN 1 84340 187 8

Cover design  Liz Wiffen
Design  XAB Design, Liz Brown
Photography  See Acknowledgments
Copy Editor  Claire Wedderburn-Maxwell
Project Editor  Serena Webb

Colour reproduction by Classic Scan Pte Ltd, Singapore
Printed and bound by Printer Trento, Italy

SAFETY NOTE
The information in this book is not intended as a substitute for
medical advice. Any person suffering from conditions requiring
medical attention, or who has symptoms that concern them,
should consult a qualified medical practitioner.

I dedicate this book to my loyal family and friends and to all
the people who have helped put it together.
(Ian Marber)

I wish to thank my parents, who brought me up to believe
that anything is possible in life, if you're prepared to apply
yourself to it.
(Vicki Edgson)

# contents

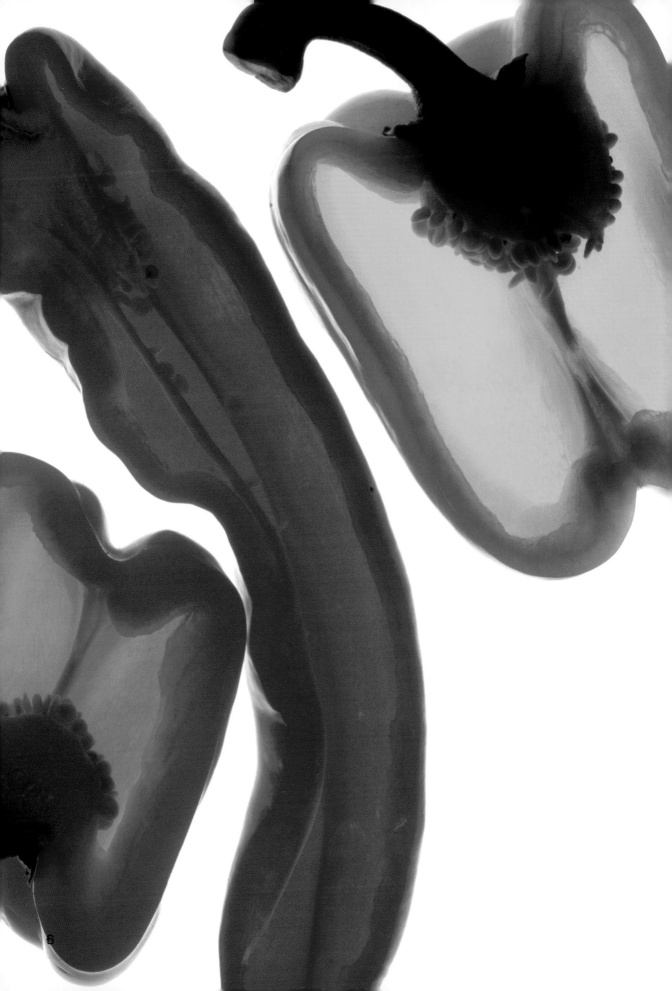

# introduction

' Rarely a day passes without yet another newspaper article being published about food and diet. What we eat has become an obsession, yet all too many people make their decisions on what to eat based solely on whether they believe that food will lead to weight gain or weight loss. But there is far more to food than that.

More than ever, we believe in the true properties and potential value of food. What you eat can have a profound effect on how you feel, and can help reduce the risk of disease, as well as promoting vitality and energy. This new and fully revised edition of *The Food Doctor* has been expanded to include information on yet more common complaints, a guide to nutrients and a new chapter on vegetarian and vegan eating.

We both hope that you will enjoy this new edition, and invite you to find out yet more at www.thefooddoctor.com. '

IAN MARBER                    VICKI EDGSON

www.thefooddoctor.com

# lifestyle questionnaire

As nutrition consultants, we regularly find that clients come to us with the same problems, the causes of which are often not immediately apparent. For some ailments, over-the-counter remedies can be tried; however, these will not address the root causes of the problem: an investigation of the client's lifestyle is needed.

Listed below are the 20 health problems most frequently described by our clients. If you have a similar problem, refer to the relevant questionnaire. If you find that you answer 'yes' to most of the questions, we show you the possible underlying causes. For example, feeling tired all the time could be put down to the pressures of work or children, but if sugar and caffeine cravings are also experienced, it could indicate an allergy or yeast infection. The common denominator for many symptoms is the health and efficiency of the gut which, in turn, is closely linked to the liver and the pancreas. Encouraging the digestive system to become more efficient helps symptoms to improve within a relatively short period of time. Look up these problems in the other chapters of this book where they are discussed more fully. Bear in mind that the causes listed here are 'possible' causes, and are not intended as a substitute for advice from your doctor.

## 1 LACK OF ENERGY/FATIGUE

### Questionnaire

- Do you feel tired all the time?
- Are you irritable and snappy?
- Does sleep leave you unrefreshed?
- Do you feel drained mid-afternoon?
- Do you often feel unwell for no apparent reason?
- Is your intake of sugar, tea and coffee high?

**Possible causes:** gut permeability and food intolerances, gut dysbiosis and yeast overgrowth, toxic metals, low blood pressure, low thyroid function, limited diet and poor blood sugar management, nutrient deficiencies.

## 2 PAIN AND INFLAMMATION

### Questionnaire

- Do you have arthritic pain in any joints or digits?
- Are any joints swollen?
- Do you have much neck, shoulder, or back pain?
- Are most of your meals fast or convenience food?
- Do you use non-prescription painkillers, such as Ibuprofen, daily?

**Possible causes:** food intolerances, gut dysbiosis and yeast overgrowth, deficiencies of essential fatty acids, auto-immune disease, thyroid imbalance, physical injury, impaired detoxification by the liver.

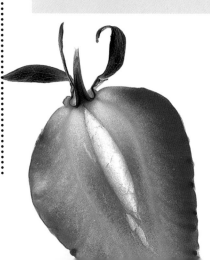

## 3 INDIGESTION

### Questionnaire

- Do you often get stomach pains after eating?
- Are you frequently constipated?
- Do your stools contain partly undigested foods?
- Do you suffer from bouts of belching?
- Do you regularly chew gum?

**Possible causes:** low level of stomach acid, lack of digestive enzymes, bacterial infections and parasites, food intolerances, gastric or duodenal ulcer, frequent use of antacids, impaired liver function.

## 4 GAS AND BLOATING

### Questionnaire

- Do you feel bloated immediately after eating?
- Is gas frequently a problem?
- Do you often get abdominal cramps?
- Are you a regular alcohol drinker?
- Do you crave sweet foods, bread, pasta, or wine?

**Possible causes:** low level of stomach acid, lack of digestive enzymes, bacterial/parasitic infections, food intolerances, poor elimination, poor food choices.

## 5 HEADACHES AND MIGRAINES

### Questionnaire

- Do you regularly take painkillers for headaches?
- Do you eat lots of chocolate or dairy foods?
- Are the above more acute at menstruation?
- Have you any food allergies?
- Do you experience digestive problems?

**Possible causes:** food intolerances, gut permeability, toxic metals, vasoconstriction attributable to smoking, alcohol, blood sugar mismanagement, postural misalignment or injury, visual impairment.

## 6 PMS

### Questionnaire

- Are your periods irregular?
- Do you experience premenstrual cramps?
- Are you irritable, intolerant, or anxious prior to menstruation?
- Do you suffer from weight gain or water retention each month?
- Do you crave sweet/starchy foods before a period?

**Possible causes:** magnesium and vitamin B6 deficiencies, poor circulation, hormonal imbalances, pituitary hormone imbalances, stress.

## 7 ANXIETY AND NERVOUSNESS

### Questionnaire

- Do you always imagine the worst?
- Do you have many fillings in your teeth?
- Were you brought up in an industrial area?
- Do you crave sugar and sweet foods?
- Do you consume soft drinks and/or caffeine daily?

**Possible causes:** toxic metals and environmental pollutants, brain chemical imbalances, amino acid imbalances, impaired liver function, food intolerances, yeast overgrowth, stress.

## 8 DEPRESSION

### Questionnaire

- Are you an irregular eater?
- Do you use food to alleviate the blues?
- Are you a heavy smoker or drinker?
- Do you lack motivation?
- Do you experience problems in sleeping?

**Possible causes:** blood sugar mismanagement, toxic metals and environmental pollutants, brain chemical imbalances, bacterial and yeast overgrowths, gut dysbiosis, food intolerances, stress, family history, recreational drug abuse.

## 9 HIGH BLOOD PRESSURE OR HIGH CHOLESTEROL LEVEL; CHEST PAIN

### Questionnaire
- Do you suffer from palpitations?
- Are you out of breath after climbing the stairs?
- Do your hands or feet tingle?
- Do you add salt during cooking and to meals?
- Are you a smoker?
- Are fried foods a major part of your diet?
- Are you more than 10 kilos (22 lb) overweight?

**Possible causes:** lack of exercise, nutritional deficiencies, diet high in saturated fat and fried foods, low thyroid function, adrenal stress, smoking, excessive alcohol consumption, high salt intake, heart disease.

## 10 DIABETES (TYPE II – MATURITY ONSET)

### Questionnaire
- Do you eat a lot of sweet snacks?
- Do you experience mood swings during the day?
- Are you frequently irrational and argumentative?
- Are you thirsty all the time?
- Do you urinate frequently?
- Are you constantly tired?

**Possible causes:** pancreatic insufficiency (lowered insulin production), high carbohydrate diet, lack of digestive enzymes, obesity, lack of exercise, impaired liver function, adrenal stress, chromium and vitamin B3 deficiencies.

## 11 INFERTILITY (male and female)

### Questionnaire
- Have you been trying to conceive for more than one year?
- Do you drink alcohol regularly?
- Are you under a lot of stress?
- Do you eat a lot of fast or convenience foods?
- Do you live in a highly polluted area?

**Possible causes:** hormonal imbalances, bacterial and parasitic infections, toxic metals and environmental pollutants, specific nutrient deficiencies (essential fatty acids, magnesium, zinc, some amino acids), food intolerances, physical obstructions.

## 12 ALLERGIES

### Questionnaire
- Do you get hayfever or a runny nose (rhinitis)?
- Do you have frequent headaches?
- After eating, do you get palpitations?
- Are you experiencing skin irritation?
- Do you crave specific foods?
- Do you often feel depressed?

**Possible causes:** gut dysbiosis and permeability, vaccinations, environmental pollution, poor liver function, imbalance of essential fatty acids, adrenal stress, low level of stomach acid, lack of digestive enzymes.

## 13 SKIN PROBLEMS

### Questionnaire
- Have you travelled abroad a lot recently?
- Is your skin irritated by heat or direct sunlight?
- Are you under a lot of stress?
- Do you regularly drink alcohol?
- Do you eat a lot of dairy or convenience foods?
- Do you eat any of the same foods every day?

**Possible causes:** food intolerances (specifically dairy, wheat and citrus), hormonal imbalances, parasitic infections, deficiencies in essential fatty acids and vitamin C, a junk-food diet.

## 14 ECZEMA AND ASTHMA

### Questionnaire
- Is your diet high in fried foods and red meat?
- Do you eat dairy produce daily?
- Are you drinking alcohol on a regular basis?
- Are you on any prescription or over-the-counter medication?

**Possible causes:** food intolerances (especially dairy, wheat and citrus), imbalance of essential fatty acids, allergy to cosmetics, cleaning agents and dust mites, diet high in saturated fats.

## 15 HYPERACTIVITY

### Questionnaire

- Do you eat a lot of sweet foods?
- Are convenience or ready meals a staple?
- Do you drink coloured soft drinks and sodas?
- Are you already on medication for hyperactivity?
- Do you regularly take aspirin?

**Possible causes:** food allergies and intolerances, sensitivity to food additives, salicylate sensitivity (aspirin-like compounds found in certain foods), deficiency in essential fatty acids, environmental pollutants and toxic metals, vaccinations.

## 16 DIARRHOEA/CONSTIPATION

### Questionnaire

- Do you suffer from alternate bouts of diarrhoea and constipation?
- Is your diet low in fruit and vegetables?
- Do you hardly ever exercise?
- Are you taking any over-the-counter painkillers?
- Are you using laxatives?

**Possible causes:** gut inflammation and permeability, diet low in fibre, lack of exercise, bacterial/parasitic infections, poor posture, smoking, high alcohol consumption, poor liver function.

## 17 COLDS, FLU AND FREQUENT INFECTIONS

### Questionnaire

- Have you recently lost someone close to you?
- Are you recovering from surgery?
- Are you frequently under stress?
- Do you consume a lot of dairy produce?
- Are you suffering from any known food or environmental allergies?

**Possible causes:** lowered immune function, adrenal stress, food intolerances and gut permeability, bacterial infections, lack of vitamins A, C and E, and zinc and selenium.

## 18 YEAST INFECTIONS AND CYSTITIS

### Questionnaire

- Do you suffer from digestive problems?
- Do you frequently eat animal products?
- Is your diet high in sugar?
- Do you suffer from mouth ulcers (canker sores)?
- Are you urinating frequently?

**Possible causes:** gut dysbiosis and permeability, bacterial infections, high-acid diet.

## 19 EATING DISORDERS AND OBESITY

### Questionnaire

- Are you afraid of food?
- Do you think about food all the time?
- Do you crave specific foods?
- Are you in the habit of weighing yourself daily?
- Are you more than 20 kilos (44 lb) overweight?
- Are you secretive about your eating habits?

**Possible causes:** imbalanced thyroid function, amino acid deficiencies, lack of zinc and vitamin B6, chromium and vitamin B3 deficiencies, too much or too little exercise, pancreatic insufficiency, poor blood sugar management.

## 20 CONCENTRATION/MEMORY LOSS

### Questionnaire

- Do you eat irregularly?
- Do you have a lot of amalgam tooth fillings?
- Are you a regular consumer of caffeinated drinks?
- Do you have food cravings?
- Are you suffering from any digestive discomfort?

**Possible causes:** toxic metals and environmental pollutants, bacterial and parasitic infections, poor blood sugar management, multiple nutrient deficiencies.

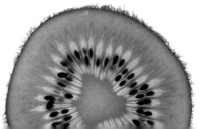

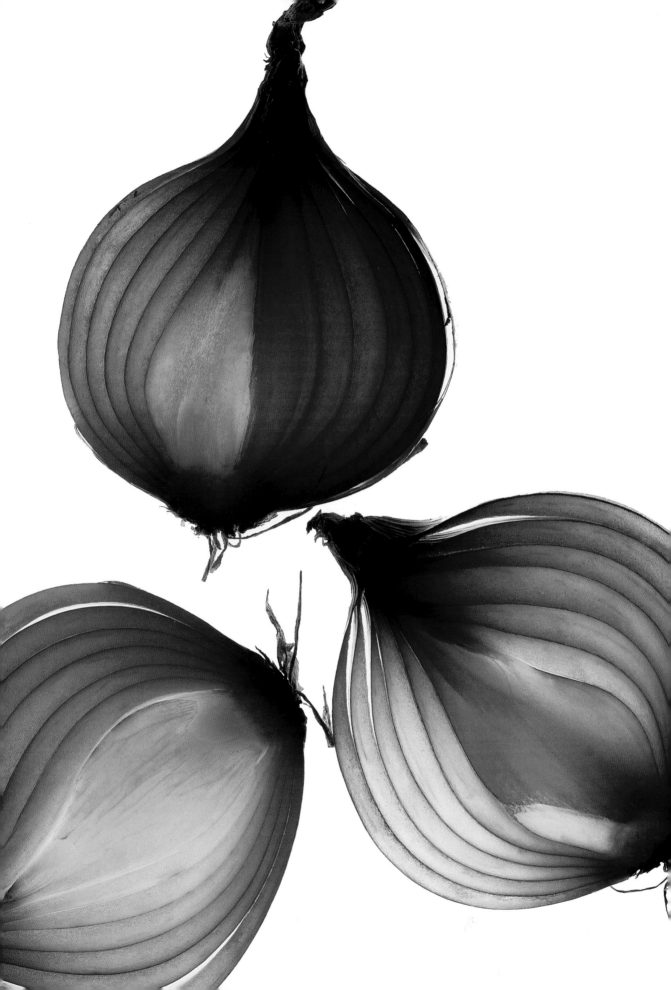

# your top 100 foods for health

Whatever your lifestyle, it's not difficult to make small changes that can have positive effects on your health. By learning more about the benefits of basic ingredients rather than relying on pre-packaged foods, you can make informed choices about what you eat. Every fruit and vegetable, as well as fish, chicken and other poultry, dairy products, legumes and grains have nutritional benefits. Variety is the key to a better-balanced diet, ensuring maximum energy, repair and immunity.

| Food | Nutrients | Benefits |
|---|---|---|
| Apples | Calcium, magnesium, phosphorus, vitamin C, beta-carotene, pectin. | Astringent, tonic. Relieve constipation, reactivate beneficial gut bacteria, reduce total cholesterol. Help remove toxins. |
| Apricots | Copper, calcium, magnesium, potassium, folic acid, vitamin C, beta-carotene, boron, iron. | Laxative, potent antioxidant, natural sweetener. Improve circulation. |
| Avocados | Iron, copper, phosphorus, potassium, beta-carotene, folic acid, vitamin B3, vitamin B5, vitamin K. High in vitamin E. | Acid–alkaline content is balanced. Easily digested, good for the blood and prevent anaemia. |
| Bananas | Potassium, tryptophan (an amino acid), vitamin C, beta-carotene, vitamin K, vitamin B6. | Promote sleep. Mild laxative. Anti-fungal, natural antibiotic. Contain pectin, which helps ulcers, lowers cholesterol, and removes toxic metals from the body. |

Fruits

Fruits

| Food | Nutrients | Benefits |
|------|-----------|----------|
| **Black-berries** | Calcium, magnesium, potassium, phosphorus, beta-carotene, vitamin C. | Tonic and blood cleanser. Relieve diarrhoea. Antioxidant. |
| **Blueberries** | Vitamin C, beta-carotene. | Laxative, blood cleanser, improve circulation, benefit eyesight, antioxidant. |
| **Cherries** | Calcium, phosphorus, vitamin C. | Antispasmodic, relieve headaches. Juice fights gout. Natural antiseptic. |
| **Cranberries** | Potassium, beta-carotene, vitamin C. | Excellent for the respiratory system. Kill bacteria and viruses in the kidneys, bladder and urinary tract. |
| **Dates** | Calcium, iron, beta-carotene, vitamin B3. | Excellent against diarrhoea and dysentery, good for problems with the respiratory system. |
| **Figs** | Calcium, magnesium, phosphorus, potassium, beta-carotene, vitamin C. | Laxative, restorative, increase vitality. Move sluggish bowels, clear toxins. One of the highest plant sources of calcium. |
| **Grapefruit** | Calcium, magnesium, potassium, vitamin C. | Contain salicylic acid, which helps arthritis. Excellent for cardiovascular system. Blood cleansing. Good for allergies and infections of the throat and mouth. |
| **Kiwi fruit** | Magnesium, phosphorus, potassium, vitamin C. | Remove excess sodium in the body. Excellent source of digestive enzymes. |

Fruits

| Food | Nutrients | Benefits |
|------|-----------|----------|
| Lemons/ Limes | Potassium, vitamin C. | Astringent, potent antiseptic, excellent for colds, coughs, sore throats. Dissolve gallstones. Anti-cancer properties. |
| Mangoes | High in beta-carotene, vitamin C. | Beneficial for kidneys, combat acidity and poor digestion. Good blood cleanser. |
| Melons | Calcium, magnesium, potassium, phosphorus, vitamin C, beta-carotene. | Excellent cleanser and rehydrator. High water content. Should be eaten on their own for maximum benefit. |
| Oranges | Calcium, potassium, beta-carotene, folic acid, vitamin C. | Stimulating, tonifying, cleansing. Internal antiseptic. Stimulate peristalsis. |
| Papayas | Calcium, magnesium, potassium, vitamin C, beta-carotene. | Excellent for aiding digestion. Anti-parasitic, anti-cancer. Soothe intestinal inflammation and gas and detoxify generally. |
| Peaches | Calcium, magnesium, phosphorus, vitamin C, potassium, beta-carotene, folic acid. | Diuretic, laxative, easily digested, alkaline. Cleansing for kidneys and bladder. |
| Pears | Calcium, magnesium, phosphorus, potassium, beta-carotene, folic acid. High in iodine. | Diuretic. High iodine content, beneficial for thyroid function. Contain pectin, which aids peristalsis and the removal of toxins. |
| Pineapples | Calcium, phosphorus, potassium, beta-carotene. | Contain bromelain, a potent digestive enzyme, scavenging bacteria and parasites; very similar to stomach acid. Not kind to teeth enamel. |

| Food | Nutrients | Benefits |
|------|-----------|----------|
| Fruits |  |  |
| **Prunes** | Calcium, phosphorus, potassium, beta-carotene, folic acid. | Laxative, containing oxalic acid. Beneficial for blood, brain and nerves. Help to lower cholesterol. |
| **Rasp-berries** | Calcium, magnesium, phosphorus, potassium, vitamin B3, vitamin C. | Help expel mucus, phlegm, toxins. Excellent for female reproductive health. Relieve menstrual cramps; however, raspberry leaf tea should not be drunk during pregnancy. |
| **Straw-berries** | Vitamin A, vitamin C, vitamin K, beta-carotene, folic acid and potassium. | Anti-cancer, antiviral, antibacterial. |
| Vegetables **Tomatoes** | Calcium, magnesium, phosphorus, beta-carotene, folic acid, vitamin C. | Contain over 90 per cent water. Antiseptic, alkaline. Raw tomatoes reduce liver inflammation. Eating large quantities can interfere with calcium absorption. |
| **Asparagus** | Phosphorus, potassium, folic acid, beta-carotene, vitamin C, vitamin K. | Contain asparagine, which stimulates the kidneys. Mild laxative, antibacterial. Caution: contains purine – avoid if you suffer from gout. |
| **Aubergine** (Eggplant) | Calcium, phosphorus, beta-carotene, folic acid. | Clean blood, prevent strokes and haemorrhages, protect arteries damaged by cholesterol. |
| **Beetroot** | Calcium, magnesium, iron, phosphorus, potassium, manganese, folic acid, vitamin C. | Excellent intestinal cleanser. Good blood builder, detoxify liver and gall bladder. |
| **Broccoli** | Calcium, magnesium, vitamin B3, vitamin B5, beta-carotene, phosphorus. High in vitamin C, folic acid. | Anti-cancer, antioxidant, intestinal cleanser, excellent source of fibre, antibiotic, antiviral (from sulphur) – stimulates liver. A perfect food. |

Vegetables

| Food | Nutrients | Benefits |
|------|-----------|----------|
| **Brussels sprouts** | Calcium, magnesium, iron, phosphorus, potassium, beta-carotene, vitamin B3, vitamin B6, vitamin C, vitamin E, folic acid. | Antioxidant, anti-cancer, antibacterial and antiviral. Support pancreatic function. Contain indoles, which protect against breast and colon cancer. Help guard against colon cancer (as does broccoli). |
| **Cabbage** | Calcium, magnesium, potassium, phosphorus, beta-carotene, folic acid, vitamin C, vitamin E, vitamin K, iodine. | Eaten raw, it detoxifies the stomach and upper colon; improves digestion. Stimulates the immune system, kills bacteria and viruses. Anti-cancer and antioxidant. |
| **Carrots** | Calcium, magnesium, potassium, phosphorus, beta-carotene. | Superb detoxifier, excellent food for the health of the liver and digestive tract. Carrots help kidney function and kill bacteria and viruses. |
| **Cauliflowers** | Calcium, magnesium, folic acid, potassium, boron, beta-carotene, vitamin C. | Help purify the blood. Good for bleeding gums, kidney and bladder disorders, high blood pressure, constipation. Anti-cancer and antioxidant. |
| **Celeriac** | Calcium, magnesium, potassium, vitamin C. | Diuretic, good for kidney stones and arthritis. Beneficial to the nervous and lymphatic systems. |
| **Celery** | Beta-carotene, folic acid, vitamin B3, sodium. | Contains coumarins, which have good anti-cancer properties. Lowers blood pressure, can help migraines. Aids digestion. Prevents fermentation. Helps arthritic joints, prevents calcium deposits. |
| **Cucumbers** | Potassium, beta-carotene. | Diuretic, laxative. Dissolve the uric acid that causes kidney and bladder stones. Help digestion. Regulate blood pressure. |
| **Fennel** | Calcium, magnesium, phosphorus, sodium, folic acid, vitamin C, potassium. Rich in phyto-oestrogens. | Anti-spasmodic, relieves intestinal cramps and stomach pain. Beneficial during the menopause. Digests fats well, useful in obesity and weight control. |

Vegetables

| Food | Nutrients | Benefits |
|------|-----------|----------|
| **Globe artichokes** | Calcium, magnesium, phosphorus, potassium, sodium, folic acid, beta-carotene, vitamin B3, vitamin C, vitamin K. | Diuretic, digestive. Contain inulin, which stimulates bacteria in the gut. Support and cleanse the liver, promote bile flow, lower cholesterol. |
| **Leeks** | Potassium, vitamin K, calcium, folic acid, vitamin A. | Cleansing, diuretic. Eliminate uric acid in gout. |
| **Lettuce** | Beta-carotene, magnesium, potassium, folic acid. | Anti-spasmodic. Contains silicon, which supports bones, joints, arteries and connective tissue. |
| **Mushrooms** | Calcium, iron, magnesium, vitamin B3, vitamin B5, folic acid, zinc. | Thin the blood, lower cholesterol. Support immune function. Shiitake mushrooms contain a potent anti-cancer element. |
| **Okra** | Calcium, magnesium, phosphorus, folic acid, vitamin B3, potassium, beta-carotene. | Soothing to the intestinal tract. Beneficial for IBS, bloating and gas. |
| **Olives** | Calcium, iron, beta-carotene. | Easily digested. Beneficial for liver and gall bladder, increasing secretion of bile. Stimulate peristalsis. |
| **Onions** | Calcium, magnesium, phosphorus, potassium, beta-carotene, folic acid, quercetin. | Antiseptic, anti-spasmodic, antibiotic. Reduce spasms in asthma. High capability for detoxifying – remove heavy metals and parasites. |
| **Palm hearts** | Beta-carotene, vitamin E. | Antibacterial, excellent for skin and hormonal health. Should be eaten in raw form (usually available in cans) and not cooked, because cooking releases toxins. |

Vegetables

| Food | Nutrients | Benefits |
|------|-----------|----------|
| Parsnips | Potassium, phosphorus, folic acid, calcium, magnesium. | Diuretic, support kidneys and spleen. Detoxify and cleanse the body. Improve bowel action. |
| Peas | Calcium, magnesium, phosphorus, B vitamins, folic acid, potassium, zinc, iron. | Good source of vegetable protein. Tone the stomach and aid liver function. |
| Peppers | Potassium, beta-carotene, folic acid, vitamin B, vitamin C. | Antibacterial, stimulant. Normalize blood pressure, improve circulatory system, boost secretion of saliva and stomach acid, help peristalsis. |
| Potatoes | Potassium, vitamin B3, folic acid, vitamin C. | Potato juice is very cleansing, benefiting the liver and muscles, and providing energy. |
| Radishes | Calcium, magnesium, potassium, phosphorus, beta-carotene, folic acid, vitamin C. | Expectorant, dissolve excess mucus or phlegm. Clear sinuses and sore throats. Aid production of digestive juices, particularly when eaten with starches. |
| Sea vegetables | Calcium, iron, potassium. Sea vegetables are seaweeds such as kelp, carrageen and samphire. | Highest source of these minerals, and excellent for cardiovascular and nervous systems. Cleanse the body of toxins, aid digestion. A perfect food for vegetarians. |
| Spinach | Beta-carotene, folic acid, potassium, iron, vitamin B6, vitamin C, calcium, magnesium. | Anti-cancer. Regulates blood pressure. Boosts the immune system. Supports bone health. |
| Spirulina | Phosphorus, potassium, sodium, vitamin B3, gamma-linoleic acid, beta-carotene. Spirulina are nutrient-rich algae available as a dry powder. Can be added to soups and vegetable juices. | Easily digested, perfect protein. Benefit cell regeneration, reverse ageing, protect kidneys from the by-products of medicines. Fight tumours. Anti-fungal and antibacterial. |

Vegetables

Herbs and spices

| Food | Nutrients | Benefits |
|------|-----------|----------|
| 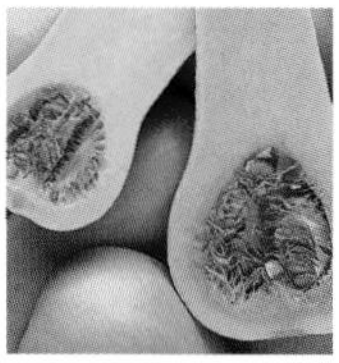 **Squash** | Calcium, magnesium, phosphorus, potassium, beta-carotene, vitamin C. | Highly alkaline, relieve acidosis of the liver and blood. Eating the seeds expels roundworms and tapeworms. |
| 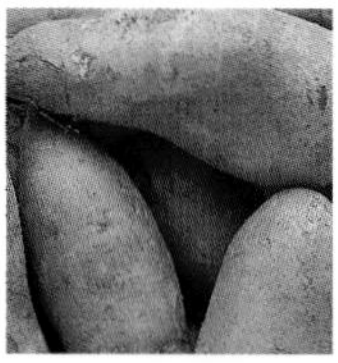 **Sweet potatoes** | Calcium, magnesium, potassium, folic acid, vitamin C, vitamin E, phosphorus, beta-carotene. | Easily digestible and highly nutritious. Excellent for inflammation of the digestive tract, ulcers and poor circulation. Detoxifying – bind to heavy metals and remove them from the body. |
| 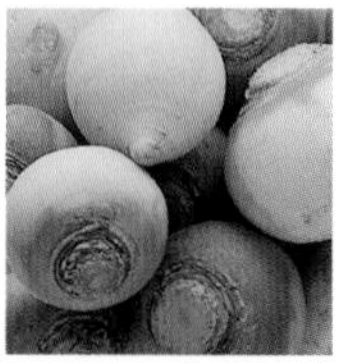 **Turnips** | Calcium, magnesium, phosphorus, potassium, folic acid, vitamin C. | Eaten raw, turnips aid digestion, and clean the teeth. Alkaline, so help purify the body. May cause gas if digestion is weak. Help clear the blood of toxins. |
| 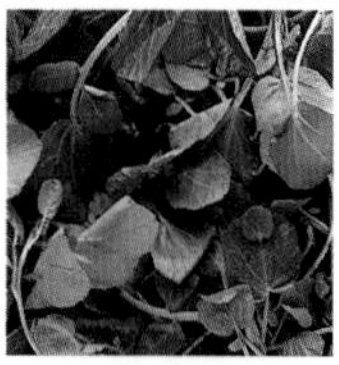 **Watercress** | Calcium, magnesium, phosphorus, potassium, vitamin C, beta-carotene. | Diuretic, breaks up kidney or bladder stones. One of the best foods for purifying the blood and relieving phlegm. High iodine content. Stimulates thyroid. |
| 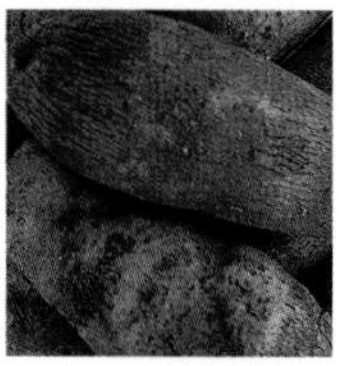 **Yams** | Calcium, magnesium, phosphorus, vitamin C, potassium, folic acid. | Anti-arthritic, anti-spasmodic, diuretic, tonifying. Bind to heavy metals to aid detoxification. Excellent for symptoms of IBS, PMS and menopause. Regulate oestrogens. |
| 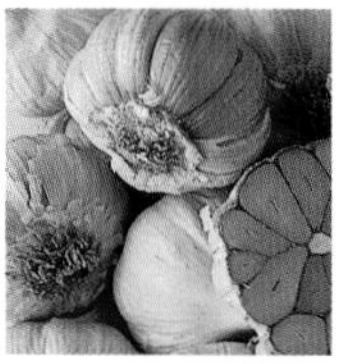 **Garlic** | Calcium, phosphorus, potassium, vitamin C. | Antibacterial, antiseptic, antiviral, decongestant. Lowers cholesterol. Nature's own antibiotic. A perfect food. |
| 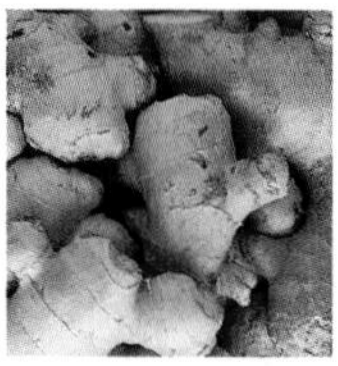 **Ginger** | Calcium, magnesium, phosphorus, potassium. | Anti-spasmodic, prevents nausea, improves circulation. Good for menstrual cramps. Excellent for convalescence. |
| 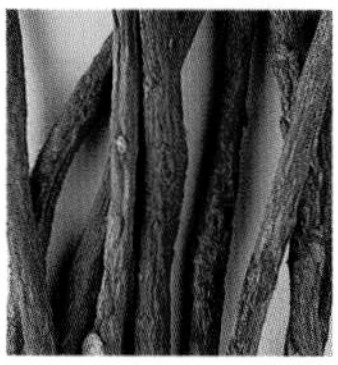 **Licorice** | Magnesium, iron, phosphorus, calcium, manganese, vitamin B3, vitamin C. | Good for adrenal function. Diuretic, laxative. Cleanses mouth and teeth. May counteract some viruses such as herpes and HIV. Assists digestion and supports the liver. |

| Food | Nutrients | Benefits |
|------|-----------|----------|
| 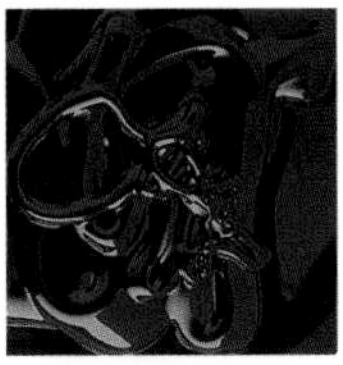 **Molasses** | Calcium, magnesium, phosphorus, potassium, manganese, B vitamins. | Contains more calcium than milk. Use in moderation. |
| 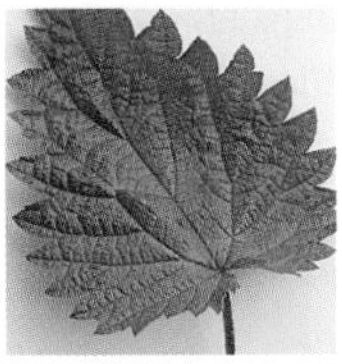 **Nettles** | Potassium, iron, vitamin C, beta-carotene. | Diuretic, anti-inflammatory, detoxifying. Nettle tea is good for gout and arthritis. |
| 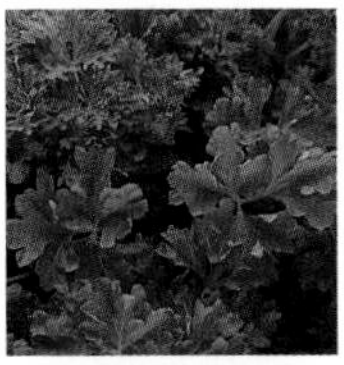 **Parsley** | Vitamin C, iron, calcium, sodium. | Cleanser, tonic, breath freshener. Alkaline. Cleanses blood, reduces coagulants in veins. Clears kidney stones. |
| 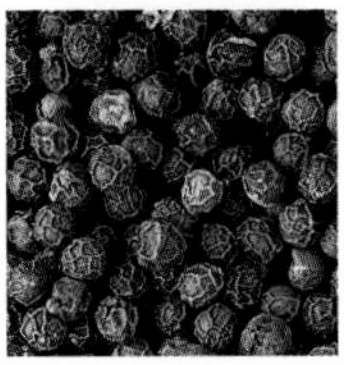 **Pepper-corns** | Calcium, magnesium, potassium, manganese, phosphorus. | Digestive stimulant, antioxidant and antibacterial. |
| 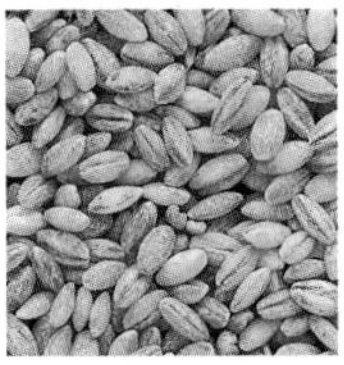 **Barley** | Potassium, magnesium, phosphorus, calcium, zinc, manganese, B vitamins, folic acid. | Soothing to the digestive tract and liver, heals stomach ulcers, lowers cholesterol. |
| 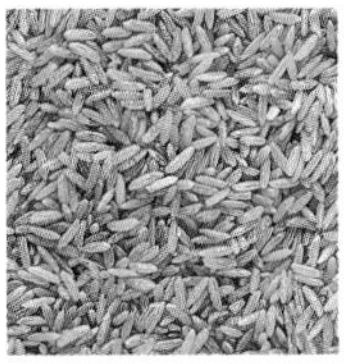 **Brown rice** | Calcium, iron, magnesium, phosphorus, potassium, zinc, manganese, vitamin B3, vitamin B5, vitamin B6, folic acid. | Calming to the nervous system, relieves depression. An energy food. Rice water is beneficial for infant colic and alleviates diarrhoea. |
| 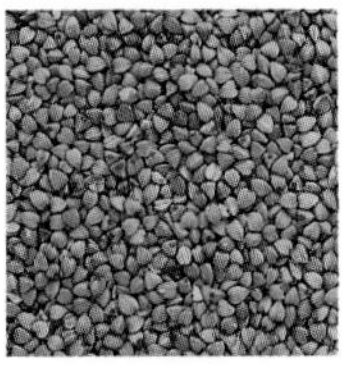 **Buckwheat** | Phosphorus, beta-carotene, vitamin C, calcium, magnesium, phosphorus, potassium, zinc, manganese, folic acid, essential amino acids. An excellent vegetable protein. | Strengthens capillaries, detoxifies. Contains all eight essential amino acids, making it a perfect vegetarian protein alternative. |
| 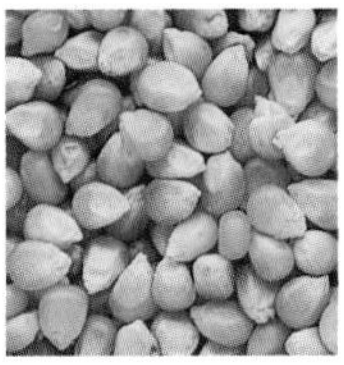 **Corn** | Iron, magnesium, potassium, zinc, vitamin B3. | Excellent food for brain and nervous system. Good for eczema. Anti-cancer food. Rich source of essential fats. |

Herbs and spices

Wholegrains

| Food | Nutrients | Benefits |
|---|---|---|
| **Millet** | Magnesium, potassium, phosphorus, vitamin B3. | Gluten-free grain, easily digestible. Highly alkaline. Rich in fibre. Low-allergenic food. |
| **Oats** | Calcium, magnesium, iron, phosphorus, manganese, vitamin B5, folic acid, silicon. | High fibre content ensures a mild laxative effect. Stimulate digestive function. Antioxidant properties. Excellent for bones and connective tissue. |
| **Quinoa** | Calcium, iron, magnesium, phosphorus, potassium, vitamin B3. | Easy to digest. Gluten-free. Lysine content is a potent antiviral agent. Contains more calcium than milk. Stimulates milk flow in breastfeeding. Perfect vegetable protein. |
| **Rye** | Calcium, iron, magnesium, phosphorus, potassium, zinc, manganese, vitamin E. | An energy food. Cleanses and renews arteries, benefits the liver, rebuilds the digestive system. |
| **Wheat** | Calcium, iron, magnesium, phosphorus, potassium, zinc, manganese, vitamin B3, vitamin B5, vitamin B6, folic acid. | Organic wholewheat (unbleached, with no chemical washing, with germ and bran left intact) stimulates the liver and cleanses toxins. |
| **Wild rice** | Iodine, selenium, vitamin E, tryptophan (an amino acid), potassium. | Excellent vegetarian source of protein. |
| **Chickpeas** | Calcium, magnesium, phosphorus, potassium, zinc, manganese, beta-carotene. High in folic acid. | Support kidney function. Digestive cleanser. Excellent source of vegetable protein. |
| **Kidney beans** | Calcium, magnesium, phosphorus, potassium, folic acid, protein. | High in fibre, cleanse the digestive tract. Increase beneficial bacteria, remove excess cholesterol. |

| Food | Nutrients | Benefits |
|------|-----------|----------|
| 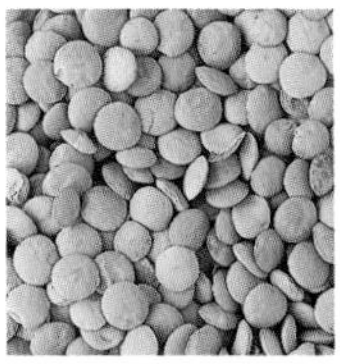 **Lentils** | Calcium, magnesium, phosphorus. Rich source of potassium, zinc, folic acid. | Good source of minerals for nearly every organ in the body. Neutralize acids produced in muscles. |
| 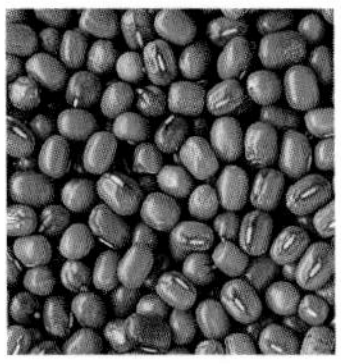 **Mung beans** | Calcium, magnesium, iron, phosphorus, potassium, zinc, vitamin B3, vitamin B5, folic acid. | Great heart and blood cleanser, excellent for detoxification. |
| 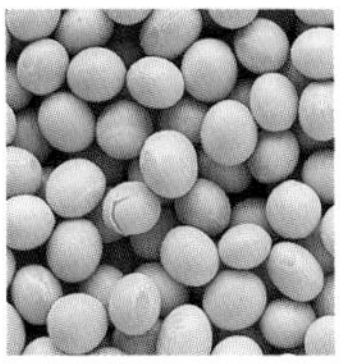 **Soya beans** | Calcium, iron, phosphorus, beta-carotene, amino acids, vitamin B3, vitamin C, omega-3 essential fatty acids, protein. | A perfect vegetarian protein. A potent phyto-oestrogen which may help prevent breast/ovarian cancers. Excellent source of lecithin to help lower cholesterol. May be used as a good alternative to cow's dairy. |
| 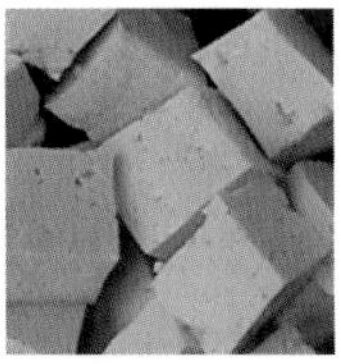 **Tofu** | Iron, amino acids, potassium, calcium, magnesium, vitamin A, vitamin K. | Perfect vegetarian source of protein. Balances hormones, anti-cancer, lowers cholesterol. |
| 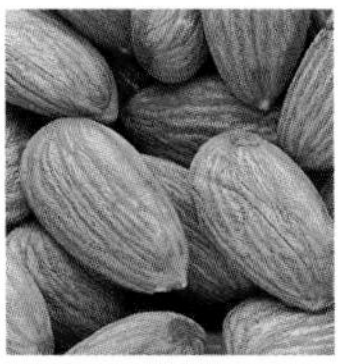 **Almonds** | Calcium, magnesium, phosphorus, potassium, zinc, folic acid, vitamin B2, vitamin B3, vitamin E. | Very alkaline, good source of protein, contain leatril (anti-cancer). Good building food for those who are underweight. |
| 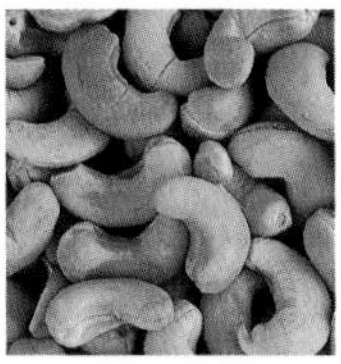 **Cashew nuts** | Calcium, magnesium, iron, zinc, folic acid. | Improve vitality, good for teeth and gums. |
| 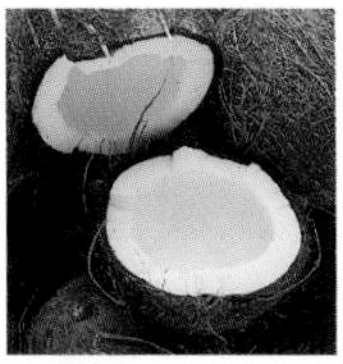 **Coconut** | Magnesium, potassium, phosphorus, zinc, folic acid, vitamin C. | Regulates thyroid function. |
| 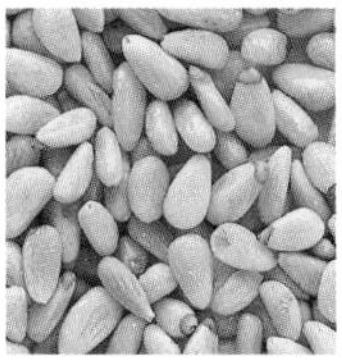 **Pine nuts** | Magnesium, potassium, zinc, B vitamins. | High in protein and essential fat. Good as a meat replacement for vegetarians. |

Pulses (Legumes)

Nuts

| | Food | Nutrients | Benefits |
|---|---|---|---|
| **Nuts** | **Walnuts** | Calcium, iron, magnesium, phosphorus, zinc, potassium, folic acid, vitamin C, vitamin E. | Strengthen the kidneys and lungs, lubricate the digestive system, improve metabolism. |
| **Seeds** | **Alfalfa** | Calcium, magnesium, potassium, manganese, sodium. | Stimulant, reduces inflammation, detoxifies, encourages sexual activity. A perfect food – but contraindicated with lupus and other autoimmune diseases. |
| | **Flaxseeds** (Linseeds) | Omega-3 and omega-6 essential fatty acids, potassium, magnesium, calcium, phosphorus, iron, vitamin B3, vitamin E. | Alleviate constipation and bloating, help eliminate toxic waste in bowels. Good for asthma. Strengthen the blood. Anti-inflammatory, anti-cancer. A perfect food. |
| | **Psyllium seeds** | Calcium, magnesium, phosphorus, potassium, zinc. | Laxative, intestinal cleanser. Relieve autotoxaemia caused by constipation and bacterial/fungal infections. |
| | **Pumpkin seeds** | Calcium, iron, magnesium, zinc, B vitamins, phosphorus, potassium, omega-6 and omega-9 essential fatty acids. | Excellent for prostate health. Remove intestinal parasites. Pumpkin seed oil is rich in omega-6 and omega-9 essential fatty acids (do not heat or the value is destroyed). |
| | **Sesame seeds** | Calcium, iron, magnesium, zinc, vitamin E, folic acid, phosphorus, potassium, copper, selenium, omega-3 and omega-6 essential fatty acids. | Strengthen heart and cardiovascular system and benefit nervous system. Contain lignans, which are antioxidants. Inhibit cholesterol absorption from the diet. |
| | **Sunflower seeds** | Vitamin A, vitamin B, vitamin D, vitamin E, vitamin K, calcium, iron, potassium, phosphorus, zinc, manganese, magnesium, omega-3 and omega-6 essential fatty acids. | A more beneficial nutrient source than most meats, eggs and cheese. Contain pectin, which removes toxins and heavy metals. Strengthen sight and sensitivity to light. A perfect food. |
| **Animal Products** | **Eggs** | Calcium, iron, manganese, zinc, B-group vitamins. First-class protein. | Good for problems with the bones and joints, boost immune system, energy food. |

**Dairy** · **Fish and seafood** · **Meat**

| Food | Nutrients | Benefits |
| --- | --- | --- |
| **Yoghurt** | Calcium, vitamin D. | Beneficial to the intestinal tract by regenerating good bacteria. Soothing, cooling. Use live organic yoghurt only, which contains acidophilus bacteria. |
| **Herring** | Omega-3 and omega-6 essential fatty acids, calcium, phosphorus. | Excellent blood cleanser, good for cardiovascular health. |
| **Mackerel** | Calcium, selenium, vitamin E, omega-3 essential fatty acids. | Maintains cardiovascular health, balances hormones. Strengthens the immune system. |
| **Oysters** | Very high in zinc. Vitamin A, vitamin B12, vitamin C, iron. | Benefit cardiovascular, immune and sexual function. |
| **Salmon** | Calcium, selenium, vitamin D, vitamin E, omega-3 essential fatty acids. | Rich source of beneficial omega-3 fish oil: good for hormonal health, skin, the immune system, bones and teeth. |
| **Tuna** | Selenium, omega-3 essential fatty acids, vitamin B12, vitamin B3. | Good for the skin, hormonal and cardiovascular systems. |
| **Chicken** | Vitamin A, vitamin B3, vitamin B6, vitamin K, sodium, potassium, magnesium. | Helps break up mucus during a cold. Mild antibiotic. |
| **Feathered game** (partridge, quail, pheasant, duck) | Selenium, full range of B vitamins, iron, zinc. | Energy-producing food: helps the body repair damage, and supports the immune system. |

# weight management

For many, the decision to alter eating habits is spurred on by a desire to lose weight. If this is your aim, we can only say to you what we say to our clients: weight loss follows healthy eating. By making good health your goal, you will have a better understanding of food and of the factors affecting weight.

The diet industry feeds directly off the pressure applied by the fashion and beauty industries, which tell us that we must look good in order to feel good. Fortunes are spent advertising 'weight-loss' foods and diet drinks. While these can help some people, we believe that ultimately, dieting doesn't work. We have both come across clients who are truly unwell, yet who will not follow a new eating plan that is designed specifically to help them recover if it involves eating foods that they consider to be 'fattening'. These clients choose to stay unwell, rather than risk any weight gain.

### Why diets don't work

Barely a week goes by without the introduction and promotion of some new fad diet – and while some weight loss will be experienced in the first few days, this is due only to the loss of fluid and not fat. Disappointment is inevitable. We have seen many clients who have followed unsafe diets – diets driven by calories rather than nutrition – which result in actual health problems. For example, a high-protein diet, over a prolonged period, can lead to bone deterioration and kidney problems; a low-fat diet may interfere with hormonal health and brain function, affecting mood and self-perception.

### Lose five pounds in five days?

Understanding what is actually lost, and what is not, is the key to safe and effective weight management. When we diet, we consume less food (fewer calories), causing the body to call upon its reserves to release glycogen, which is then used for energy. This glycogen, stored in the liver and lean muscle tissue, is held in a water base. The weight loss we experience in the early stages of a diet is simply a loss of fluid. This is the basis of the hollow promises behind diets that advertise themselves as a way of losing five pounds in five days. Yes, you do lose weight in terms of fluid loss, but there is no actual body fat loss, so the effect is temporary. If this approach is maintained for an extended period, the body perceives the relatively lower intake of food as potential starvation, so it holds on to whatever food or drink is consumed for fuel and glycogen replacement. This accounts for the dieting 'plateau' familiar to many habitual dieters who discover that, despite not eating very much, they still do not lose weight.

### Yo-yo dieting – the thyroid disrupter

Yo-yo dieters are people who spend years trying one diet after another. They are imprisoned in an eternal treadmill of losing weight, gaining weight, losing it again and, inevitably, gaining more. The frustration that this causes them is enormous, frequently bringing with it problems of depression, low self-esteem and even hormonal disruption.

The speed at which we burn up our food to convert it into energy (our metabolic rate) is governed by the thyroid gland, located at the base of the throat. This gland is essential for energy production, dictating how we feel on a day-to-day basis. Yo-yo dieting confuses the delicate balance of hormones that are fed to and from the thyroid, resulting in a slower metabolic rate. The result of this more sluggish metabolic rate is that the thyroid slows down and resets the storage levels of glycogen in the body – holding on to it rather than releasing it – making weight loss impossible. In fact, as your thyroid function is disturbed and your metabolic rate falls, weight gain actually increases. Nutrients that are important for thyroid function include selenium, which is found in shellfish, sunflower seeds, sesame seeds, Brazil and cashew nuts, potassium found in fresh fruits and vegetables, and iodine, which is found in sea vegetables.

### Stress

Two hormones released in times of stress are cortisol and DHEA (see pages 74–75). Stress alters the balance of the hormones and can encourage fat storage even when food intake is restricted. The dieter cannot lose weight, and dieting itself becomes a stress factor.

### Allergies and intolerances

Sometimes we develop an intolerance towards foods that we eat every day. When an intolerance has developed, the body will hold on to fluids to protect any potentially vulnerable areas, such as the intestinal tract. This water retention causes puffiness and weight gain.

If someone is intolerant to wheat, merely eating a bowl of cereal (granola) and a piece of toast in the morning, a sandwich for lunch, a mid-afternoon biscuit, and a pasta dish in the evening will almost guarantee weight gain, because over 50 per cent of the day's food has contained wheat. Wheat has the effect of reducing metabolism and slowing the body down. We have found that by cutting wheat out of their diet, our clients have experienced increased energy levels, decreased tissue puffiness and a reduction in weight. If you suspect a food intolerance, keep a food diary (see pages 32–33) – it will highlight how frequently you are consuming the same foods.

**Blood sugar imbalance**

We have found virtually everyone who finds it difficult to lose weight has a marked blood sugar imbalance. Resolving this hormonal imbalance is the first step to true fat loss. It also reduces inflammation, improves mood, concentration and energy levels and eliminates food cravings.

There is no substitute for fresh, colourful fruit and vegetables. The nutrients they contain support the thyroid gland and maintain a healthy metabolic rate, while their fibre content helps to remove excess fats from the body. It is best to eat fruit and vegetables raw, since cooking can destroy fibre and nutrients.

Surprisingly, we need fats to help maintain healthy weight levels. The essential fatty acids found in nuts, seeds, oily fish and olive oil are all vital for the movement of stored fats out of the adipose tissues, an important process in weight management. All cells in the body have a fatty layer that protects them from potential damage, as well as allowing nutrients in and waste matter and toxins out. This fatty layer is made up from essential fatty acids, which cannot be manufactured in the body and must be derived from the diet. If the intake of essential fatty acids is inadequate, the cell walls become more rigid, preventing toxins, such as stored fats, from leaving. The fat becomes denser and more difficult to shift as time goes on. So to get rid of fat and cellulite, eat essential fatty acids. For this reason, oily fish such as sardines, mackerel, herring, tuna, pilchards and salmon, which are rich in essential fatty acids, should be major

**Making the right choices – a good daily menu**

Forget your preconceptions and refer to the chart below to see how a typical day's meals can be balanced, varied and delicious! These are just a few examples from the recommendations we make to our clients. (See pages 130–155 for recipes.)

## breakfast

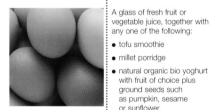

A glass of fresh fruit or vegetable juice, together with any one of the following:

- tofu smoothie
- millet porridge
- natural organic bio yoghurt with fruit of choice plus ground seeds such as pumpkin, sesame or sunflower
- sugar-free cornflakes or muesli (granola) with rice milk
- scrambled or poached eggs with tomatoes and mushrooms

## mid-morning snack

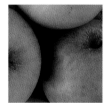

Choose one of the following:

- apple or pear with cottage cheese
- palmful of pumpkin seeds, almonds or walnuts
- half an avocado
- organic blue corn chips and low-fat houmous

## lunch

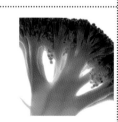

- Vegetable soup and a la[...] leafy salad plus four raw[...] vegetables from this list:

  broccoli, shredded cabbage, grated carrots or pumpkin, raw beetroo[...] mushrooms, spring (green) onions, radishes, cauliflower, peas, sweetcorn.

  *Together with one of:*
- cottage cheese
- a piece of lean chicken breast (no skin)
- a can of tuna fish, sardin[...] or salmon
- grilled fish with steamed vegetables

  *Plus:*
- some fruit, such as a banana, an apple, a few berries, tinned cherries (syrup- and sugar-free)

protein sources for anyone following a weight-management programme. For vegetarians, good sources of essential fatty acids are seeds, such as linseeds, pumpkin, sunflower and sesame, and cold-pressed oils made from them. Olive oil may also be used in moderation.

Regular exercise has many benefits for the body, and helps to maintain a healthy balance of blood sugar levels. Increasing exercise levels can be difficult when many of us tend to lead sedentary

yourself today. To aid weight loss, skin brushing should be carried out all over the body on a daily basis, to stimulate lymphatic drainage, and help to break down the stored fatty deposits. Use a natural bristle brush, rather than one with synthetic fibres, and brush the skin in sweeping strokes toward the centre of the body.

The healthy eating chart below is an example of how you can arrange your daily diet to balance your blood sugar levels, increase your vitality and

## Surprisingly, we need fats to help maintain healthy weight levels. Essential fatty acids are the good guys, helping to move stored fats out of adipose tissues.

lives. For some, sustaining impetus may involve joining a gym for workouts and exercise classes; for others, taking a daily walk or walking to work three days a week is more easily achieved. Don't procrastinate – make the commitment to

promote all-round good health, while addressing weight management. Follow the principle of combining some protein with carbohydrate at each meal, to ensure maintenance of blood sugar levels and prevent food cravings.

### mid-afternoon snack

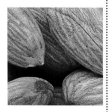

Choose one of the following:

- a piece of fruit such as an orange, a small bunch of grapes or a plum
- a palmful of mixed nuts and seeds
- two oatcakes with tahini, guacamole or avocado dip

### dinner

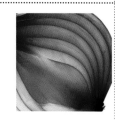

A serving of a primary protein, such as:

- fish, turkey or chicken with at least three vegetables and brown or wild rice
- rice or noodles with stir-fried chicken
- tofu and mixed vegetable stir-fry, including red peppers, carrots, French beans, mangetout or sugar snap peas, ginger, onions, mushrooms

### bedtime snack

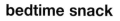

Choose one of the following:

- cottage cheese and two oatcakes
- a banana
- rice cake with low-fat houmous or nut spread (unsalted and sugar-free)

# food allergies and intolerances

Allergic reactions are now quite common. Many more of us experience allergies than people did fifty years ago. This rise can be attributed to the increase in environmental pollution, the use of pesticides and the abundance of other chemicals we use or are exposed to in our everyday lives. It is estimated that we are subjected to approximately 3,000 different chemicals every year – so it is no wonder that allergies are on the increase.

Every day, our immune systems are challenged by the chemicals we ingest in food and drinks, and the potentially toxic substances we inhale. This constant battle causes the liver to become overloaded, consequently making allergic reactions more prevalent.

In Britain, the most common food groups that people react to are wheat, dairy products, citrus fruits and eggs. In terms of human evolution, wheat is a relatively new food, having only been farmed for the last 10,000 years. It is not clear whether wheat intolerance is due to man's lack of adaptation to the grain, or if the pesticides, herbicides and chemical processes involved in preparing the grains are behind it. Wheat-based foods often form the major part of the Western daily diet, so it is possible that lack of variety may be the cause of the problem.

Gluten allergy or intolerance is a more severe form of grain allergy, and can be caused by oats, wheat, rye and barley. Those who suffer from coeliac disease (see page 91) are unable to tolerate any of these grains. In severe cases,

gluten allergy can become life-threatening as the gluten erodes the delicate lining of the digestive tract and prevents the absorption of the essential nutrients.

### When is an allergy not an allergy?

There is some confusion about allergies and intolerances. While their effects are similar, their causes are different. An allergy is defined as an immediate reaction to any stimulus, causing the immune system to produce antibodies to attack the offending molecule.

An intolerance is a delayed reaction (often not manifesting itself for several days) that causes a wide variety of symptoms, often seemingly unrelated. The chart on page 31 illustrates these differences.

In addition, many symptoms are not obviously connected to food intolerance. The range of reactions is so wide that they are often attributed to causes other than food intolerance. Such symptoms include depression, joint pain, swollen eyes, sallow, pale and/or dry skin, 'brain

## Allergy or intolerance?

There are subtle differences between a food allergy and a food intolerance. The body's reactions to a suspect food help to determine a diagnosis. To ascertain whether you have an allergy or an intolerance, check the chart below.

|  | allergy | intolerance |
| --- | --- | --- |
| **reaction time** | immediate | delayed |
| **causes** | histamine and antibodies (IgE) | antibodies (IgG) |
| **symptoms** | hives (urticaria), rashes, swelling, vomiting, palpitations, blushing, sudden tiredness | itching, raised pulse, fatigue, water retention, muscle soreness, dark circles under the eyes, headaches, migraines, diarrhoea, IBS |

fog' (difficulty in concentrating and thinking clearly), shallow breathing, constipation and/or diarrhoea, mouth ulcers (canker sores), runny nose, indigestion, skin rashes, bags and/or shadows under eyes and bed-wetting in children.

### The genetic factor

Although it is common to find allergies in children of parents who have a history of allergic problems, it does not always follow that every such child will be susceptible. The evidence indicates that children of parents who have had asthma, eczema or hayfever (atopic allergies) will have an increased susceptibility, particularly if both parents are sufferers. The fault seems to lie in the genes that determine the suppression of the release of IgE, a chemical substance in the body which is one of the mediators of the acute, instant inflammatory response to specific allergens. However, genes are not the only cause of allergy. For example, identical twins do not necessarily develop the same allergies, which indicates that other external factors, such as environmental, bacterial or viral components, may also play a part in an individual's likelihood of developing allergies.

### Digestion and allergies

Approximately 70 per cent of the body's immune system lies in the digestive tract, making this area highly reactive to troublesome foods and substances. One of the most disruptive problems for the intestines is when an overgrowth of *Candida albicans* occurs.

**nutrition know-how**

If you always have a sandwich for lunch, ensure that the type of bread and its fillings are rotated daily to prevent intolerances brought on by a repetitive diet. Try rye, wholegrain or ciabatta bread with a chicken, tuna, cheese or salad filling.

Although candida is an organism that is normally found in the gut, when the immune system is compromised, candida may get out of control and become a problem. When this happens, the candida becomes invasive, burrowing its way through the intestinal wall and creating holes and spaces in an otherwise well-guarded barrier wall. The holes and spaces allow food particles, which would not normally pass into the bloodstream, to cause immune responses there. This is a typical cause of headaches and food-intolerance-related migraines.

### Dealing with allergies and intolerances

A healthy digestive tract and an efficient immune system are essential for alleviating or preventing allergies and intolerances. Identifying trigger foods and other substances is the first step to tackling the problem. Therefore, working closely with a nutrition consultant is one of the most productive ways of approaching the subject of food allergies.

Symptomatic problems in children can often be rapidly relieved by eliminating certain trigger foods. For example, in cases of hyperactivity or attention deficit hyperactivity disorder (ADHD), the simple removal of foods that include additives and colourings often has immediate positive effects.

In adults, many long-term health problems, not previously associated with food interactions, can often be banished permanently by following exclusion programmes devised with a nutrition consultant. Eating foods in season and rotating foods daily can also help eliminate many minor food intolerances.

### Allergy testing

Many foods irritate both the digestive tract and the body as a whole. There are a variety of different types of tests that can be carried out to determine allergies, ranging from a skin-prick test to a full blood test to measure the antibody reaction caused by individual foods. The results of these tests are not always conclusive, since false positives as well as false negatives often appear. Many clients come to us with lengthy lists of foods they cannot eat. Upon further examination and investigation, we often discover that they have a compromised digestive tract function, which is causing the numerous food intolerances. To overcome this, we address the health of the digestive tract, in particular the integrity of the gut wall, and advise measures to promote its well-being. These measures usually overcome many of the food intolerance reactions, allowing our clients to enjoy their favourite foods again.

### Food diaries

In our experience, keeping a food diary that details all your food and liquid intake, and subsequent symptoms, is a very accurate method of pinpointing those foods that are causing problems. You can also keep a record of your emotional reactions to foods. For example, some people may find that within 24 hours of eating

## Anaphylactic shock

For some people, a single food could prove life-threatening if they are allergic to it and the reaction is not spotted immediately and treated appropriately. Such extreme reactions are likely to occur within minutes of consuming a food and can be recognized by the symptoms opposite.

- Closing up of the throat and nasal passages

- Inability to breathe

- Anxiety

- Panic attack

- Acute swelling of any part or all of the face and neck

tomatoes they experience joint pain, water retention and irritability; others may be vulnerable to bread and pasta, suffering reactions such as depression, headaches or sneezing.

However, if you suspect a food intolerance, it is advisable to let a qualified nutrition consultant or allergy specialist decipher your food diary. If delayed reactions are prevalent, intolerances may not be easy to determine.

### Anaphylactic shock

Anaphylactic shock is an extreme, dangerous and possibly life-threatening reaction to an antigen. Peanuts are well known for their potential to cause anaphylactic shock: many food products now carry warnings that they contain peanuts or other nuts, which may cause an allergic reaction in susceptible people. Shellfish are another major culprit behind this type of reaction, although no warning labels currently appear on such foods. Bee and wasp stings may also cause anaphylactic shock. If anaphylactic shock occurs, take the patient to

hospital immediately as they may need an adrenalin (epinephrine) injection. Check with the patient, as some sufferers carry their own injection with them. If swelling is severe, put a straw in their mouth to aid breathing

### Total toxic overload

There are those who find that they have become apparently intolerant to 'almost everything'. This is usually due to a severe gut dysbiosis, where the intestinal tract has become so inflamed that rogue food particles can pass through into the bloodstream unchecked. It is vital to address the digestive problems first, and allow the inflammation to settle.

It is also possible that the liver has become overburdened if a high intake of sugar, alcohol or prescription drugs has been consumed over a prolonged period. If the liver is overtaxed, many food-intolerance-type symptoms will present themselves, and it is essential to follow a liver-support programme. Consult a nutritionist for a personal programme.

# cooking methods

Cookery is both an art form and a pleasure. If it is done well, the look and flavour of many foods is enhanced. However, as soon as the food is subjected to heat, its nutrient level can diminish. While we recommend eating as many raw foods as possible (where it is safe to do so), we know that this does not suit everyone. We need to establish a balance between flavour and nutrient value.

Cooking changes the internal make-up of foods, making them more digestible and available for use by the body. In some cases, however, cooking can damage food to such an extent that it is turned into a potential carcinogen. For example, frying oils alters their chemical structure, rendering them harmful to vulnerable body tissue such as the cardiovascular system (see The Heart and Circulation, pages 120–135).

Some methods of cooking and preparing foods are better than others for preserving the nutrient and water levels. Vitamin C and all the B group of vitamins are water-soluble, and can easily dissolve and be lost into the cooking water or juices during intense cooking.

### Steaming

Steaming foods is perhaps the most efficient way of preserving their nutrient content. Bring a little water to the boil and place the food (usually vegetables or fish) in a steamer above the bubbling water. The steam will cook the food in just a few minutes. Dense vegetables such as carrots and broccoli usually take five minutes or so, while leaves such as spinach take less than a minute to cook. The vegetables are left *al dente* (an Italian expression, meaning they remain firm) after steaming, retaining their vivid colours, fibrous structure and nutrient content.

Steaming fish usually takes about ten minutes and preserves the delicate 'good' fats that most fish contains, as well as the water-soluble B vitamins. Fish can be steamed over water flavoured with ginger, lemon juice or fragrant herbs – an excellent way to enhance its flavour.

### Boiling

Boiling foods, especially vegetables, is the best way of making them dull and lifeless, with little nutrient content. It has been said that if vegetables such as carrots are boiled for ten minutes, the water contains more vitamin C than the carrots.

As a rule of thumb, remember that boiling vegetables destroys approximately 40 per cent of B vitamins and 70 per cent of vitamin C. The greater the amount of water in the pan, the greater the nutrient loss. This loss is further heightened when the vegetables are cut into small pieces, as a greater surface area is exposed to the water and the heat, and this can further diminish nutrient levels.

In many countries, it is common to add salt to the water when boiling vegetables. This is unnecessary: most people's diets are already too high in salt. Salt upsets the body's own sodium–water balance, as well as the heart

damaging. Although the food is cooked quickly, the extreme heat depletes the nutrients and disturbs the sensitive oils contained in foods such as oily fish. Cooking oils all have what is known as a 'smoke point': the temperature at which the oil burns. Each oil has a different smoke point – as oils are heated towards their smoke point their chemical structure is altered creating an abundance of free radicals. These free radicals are atoms that damage the body –

## Both deep and shallow frying produce foods that are palatable and attractive, yet potentially damaging.

muscle's natural rhythm. All fruit and vegetables naturally contain some sodium, and it is usually only palates that have been numbed by excessive stimulants, alcohol and sugars that crave added salt. (See page 125 for more information on salt and the heart.) So, if you are boiling food, do so for the minimum length of time, using only a small quantity of water, to preserve maximum nutrient content. Better still, steam it instead.

### Frying
Both deep and shallow frying produce foods that are palatable and attractive, yet potentially

they are involved in the initiation of cancer, in heart disease (see Arteriosclerosis and Atherosclerosis, pages 126–127) and premature ageing. Free radicals can be countered by eating foods rich in antioxidants (see Heart Nutrition, page 132). However, antioxidants are easily damaged by the high temperatures involved in frying. Browning foods by frying them, or worse still, letting them burn a little, is known to be carcinogenic. Even the smoke from frying

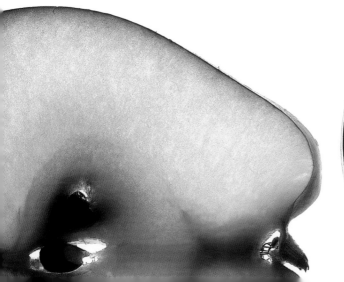

foods can be dangerous – cooks who fry food on a frequent basis have a higher risk of lung and throat cancer than those who do not.

Vitamins that are soluble in water (B and C) and fat (D, A, K and E) are lost during shallow and deep frying. Frying meat or poultry decreases its vitamin B content by as much as 30 per cent.

### Stir-frying

While stir-frying foods in a wok is always seen as the healthy alternative to deep or shallow frying, it is nonetheless still frying. Nutrients may be lost and fats are chemically altered.

However, the quantity of oil used is minimal in comparison, and the food cooks fast, because the wok ensures an even distribution of heat. If the food is cooked quickly and moved around all the time, damage is minimized.

Try adding a tablespoon of water and one of soy sauce to the oil as it heats. The liquid will stop the oil from burning, reducing the quantity of free radicals formed, and as it evaporates it will provide some steam to help cook the food. Best of all, part-cook the food in advance (steaming is best) and use the wok to finish the food.

### Microwaving

Microwaving food causes the water molecules present in the food to vibrate, and this movement creates the heat which cooks the food. The microwaves bounce off the oven walls and into the food. Nutrient levels of vegetables remain reasonably high after microwaving, probably due to the short cooking time – which is the main advantage of this

cooking method. However, nutrients are still lost, so steaming vegetables is a preferable method of cooking.

One of the biggest problems with this cooking method is the type of food that is generally cooked in microwave ovens. Processed 'ready meals' contain sugar, salt and often hydrogenated fats – all of which can be harmful to the body. In addition, when they are microwaved, these foodstuffs are the most susceptible to certain molecular changes. This change in the molecular structure can lead to free-radical damage.

### Stewing and soup-making

Cooking by stewing utilizes an extended simmering process. Stewing foods, or making casseroles and soups, ensures that the cooking liquid is served and eaten as well as the original food, so we benefit from the nutrients that are transferred into the water.

The advantage of stewed foods is that they are cooked slowly, usually at temperatures below boiling point. As vitamin and mineral loss increases with temperature, this method does not disturb the nutrient level greatly. Stewing also makes protein foods more digestible, as the fibres in the food are broken down, rendering them easier for us to absorb.

Some fruits actually benefit from stewing. For example, the enzymes in prunes are freed during this slow and gentle cooking method. Stewing fruits intensifies the taste of the natural sugar content so the flavour is best balanced with a little unsweetened live bio yoghurt.

## Roasting

Roasting meats, poultry and vegetables is a popular way to prepare foods and is an age-old cooking method in the West. The fat content of the food is relatively undisturbed, as long as the oven isn't too hot. However, if fats are allowed to burn, they become potentially carcinogenic. The browning that is synonymous with roasting is due to carbohydrates, in the form of sugars, reacting to the heat.

Some water-soluble vitamins, such as vitamin C and B-complex vitamins, are inevitably lost during roasting. It is estimated that approximately 25 per cent of B vitamins are lost during roasting, although the longer the food is cooked, the greater the vitamin loss. The same is true of temperature – the higher the temperature, the greater the nutrient loss.

## Barbecuing

A summer barbecue is always popular. The foods that are traditionally cooked on barbecues are the protein foods, meat and fish. Many people prefer to eat them slightly burnt on the outside. However, burnt food has the potential to be carcinogenic – when it comes into direct contact with the throat and digestive tract it damages cells, leading to an increase in harmful free radicals.

To minimize damage from barbecued foods, ensure that the barbecue is very hot – the coals should be white-hot and glowing, with no flames. Avoid using firelighters – foods cooked directly in their flame may become coated with the chemicals contained in the firelighters. Because of the intense heat that the food is subjected to, barbecued foods all too often appear cooked on the outside but are found to be raw in the centre. For this reason it is advisable to part-cook food in the oven first, then use the barbecue to finish the process.

## Raw food

This is by far the best way to benefit from all the available nutrients. We are not suggesting that you eat meat or grains raw, simply that you eat some raw vegetables, fruit, nuts or seeds every day. The benefit of raw foods is that they contain their own digestive enzymes, which lessen the demand on the pancreas and cells of the intestinal lining to produce these enzymes. They are also abundant sources of fibre, which encourages the removal of toxic waste and excess cholesterol from the body.

If your food usually comes with the instruction 'pierce film several times', we encourage you to set aside a little more time for cooking and eating, whenever possible. Turn to page 146 to find some suggestions for healthy, nutritious meals. Most of our recipes are quick, simple and require minimal fuss, proving that good food can be prepared in minutes – but with positive effects that last a lifetime.

**nutrition know-how**
Marinating barbecue food in olive oil (which is rich in vitamin E) before cooking offers some protection against damage by the free radicals let loose by the barbecue process.

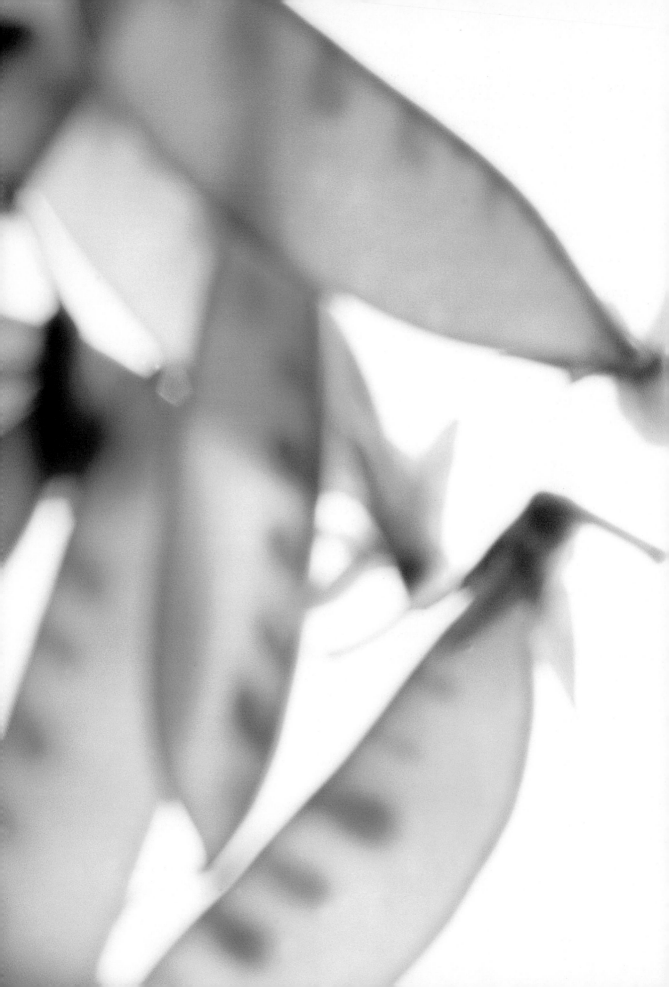

# vegetarian and vegan eating

There are many different reasons why people decide to follow a vegetarian or vegan style of eating. Vegetarians avoid eating meat and fish but do allow eggs and dairy products in their diet. Vegans, however, abstain from the consumption of any animal produce including meat, fish, eggs and dairy products, and in some cases avoid using any animal by-products, including honey, leather and wool.

Some people turn to these types of diets for health reasons. Vegetarian diets are very beneficial for those who have a high risk of cardiovascular disease since omitting red meat can greatly reduce saturated fat and cholesterol intake. The vegan diet is also believed to be beneficial to anyone suffering from cancer as some animal products contain arachidonic acid, a substance that may fuel cancer cells.

For others, the switch is for more humane or ethical reasons. Whatever the reason, these popular styles of eating, if carried out correctly, can have many benefits for both the animal world and human health.

## Understanding protein requirements

Following a balanced vegetarian and vegan diet can be a wonderful and healthy way of eating. What you need to remember is that you are seriously restricting the intake of one major food group – protein. On average, an adult requires 0.8 grams of protein per kilogram of body weight each day. Being rich in protein, animal products are an efficient way to ensure daily requirements are met. Choosing to follow a diet that contains only plant foods, which contain a lower percentage of protein, means you need to be more aware of where your daily protein requirements will be coming from.

## What are amino acids?

During digestion, enzymes break down the protein content of the food you have eaten into polypeptides, then dipeptides, then peptides, and finally into the smallest units of protein – amino acids. There is a total of 22 amino acids, and over half of these can be synthesized by your body.

Once absorbed, these amino acid units can have sections swapped or replaced to convert them into other amino acids, or they can be joined together in long chains of specific numbers, sequences and varieties to form the types of protein that you need. One way to think of them is as building blocks that can be combined to create different shapes and structures.

Out of the 22, there are eight essential amino acids. These are special in the sense that your body cannot generate or synthesize them from other amino acids. The only way your body can obtain these eight essential building blocks is from your diet.

### The essential amino acids

- Isoleucine
- Leucine
- Lysine
- Methionine
- Phenylalanine
- Threonine
- Tryptophan
- Valine

### Protein combining

Proteins are classified into two groups – complete proteins and incomplete proteins. Complete or quality proteins are rich in all the essential amino acids; these proteins include all animal products – meat, fish, eggs and dairy. Incomplete proteins, which include all plant foods, are lacking in one or more of the essential amino acids. For example, cereal (granola) grains are lacking in lysine, rice is lacking in methionine and threonine, pulses (legumes) are missing methionine and tryptophan, corn is lacking tryptophan and threonine and soya beans are missing methionine.

To enable your body to have all the necessary ingredients to generate every type of body protein and to repair and generate new body cells and tissues, a daily intake of all the essential amino acids needs to be achieved.

How do you make sure that your body gets a full intake of the eight essential amino acids whilst being a vegetarian or vegan? It's easy – you 'protein combine'. We know that pulses (legumes), wholegrains, nuts, seeds and lentils all contain different essential amino acids. Protein combining involves eating a combination of two or more plant proteins in one meal so that the full spectrum of essential amino acids is achieved. For example, eating a vegetable curry with brown rice and lentil dahl; peanut butter on rye toast or a stir-fry with tofu and cashew nuts would supply the full range of proteins.

By combining your plant foods you can increase the quality of your protein by at least 50 per cent, enabling your body to receive the full spectrum of essential amino acids. Another really easy way to increase your intake of essential amino acids is to add a heaped teaspoonful of mixed ground sesame, flax, hemp, sunflower and pumpkin seeds to your breakfast cereal (granola) or salads. As seeds and nuts are relatively high in protein compared to other plant foods they are an important component of vegetarian and vegan diets.

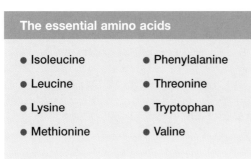

## Top Vegetarian Protein Foods

- Brown rice
- Cottage cheese
- Eggs
- Lentils

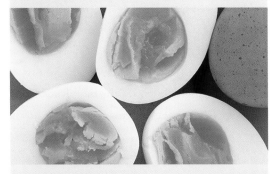

- Natural bio yoghurt
- Nuts
- Pulses (Legumes)
- Quinoa

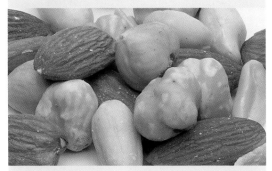

- Quorn
- Seeds
- Tempe
- Tofu

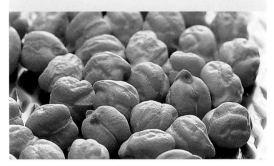

## Top Vegan Protein Foods

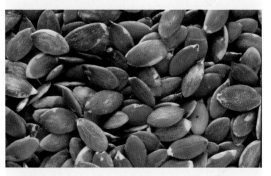

- Brown rice
- Lentils
- Nuts
- Pulses (Legumes)

- Quinoa
- Quorn
- Seeds
- Soya cheese

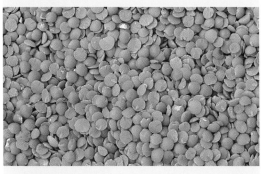

- Soya yoghurt
- Tempe
- Tofu

41

### Optimum vegetarianism and veganism

It is very easy in this day and age to become an unhealthy vegetarian or vegan. Vegetarians who rely on cheese as their major source of protein can become stuck in a rut; by eating sandwiches, pizzas, pasta and cheese-based convenience foods they will probably start to show signs of poor eating.

If you end up eating a stodgy, starchy carbohydrate- and cheese-based diet then be warned, weight gain may be just around the corner. Being a healthy vegetarian or vegan means being knowledgeable about protein combining and having a diet full of freshly prepared or home-cooked food. Even vegetarians and vegans have to make sure they are eating adequate daily levels of fresh fruits and vegetables.

### The significance of iron and B12

Iron and B12 are both important nutrients that are needed for the production of haemoglobin. This component of red blood cells acts as a transport system carrying oxygen in the blood and delivering it to cells all over the body. Oxygen is then used by the cells to generate the energy required to drive all metabolic processes.

Red meat, poultry and fish are all rich sources of both iron and B12, but since both vegetarian and vegan diets are lacking in these, care has to be taken to ensure dietary requirements are met.

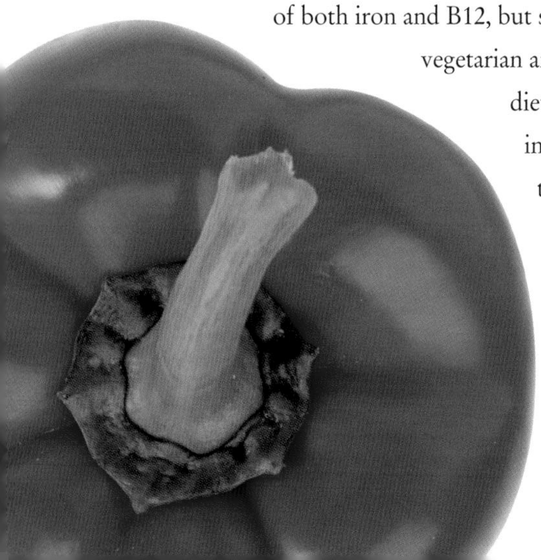

### Pale and anaemic

Iron is stored in the liver and muscles, whilst B12 is stored in reasonable quantities within the body. However, B12 levels often deplete after three to four years, whilst iron stores run out after approximately seven to eight years. This is why many vegetarians and vegans suffer from anaemia.

### Food first

Ensuring a regular intake of the foods shown opposite will prevent depletion.

Topping up with iron and B12 supplements every year will ensure that your body stores don't become depleted. We suggest you don't take iron sulphate, as this form of iron is well renowned for its digestive side-effects including constipation, bloating and abdominal pain. Go for a gentler and more absorbable form of iron such as iron fumarate. Additionally, sublingual forms of B12 are easily absorbed. Both supplements can be found at your local health food shop.

### Symptoms of anaemia

- Fatigue
- Breathlessness
- Vertical ridges in nails
- Pale skin
- Headaches
- Dizziness
- Depression
- Muscle pains
- Exhaustion after light exercise

## Top sources of Iron

- Spinach
- Parsley
- Bean sprouts

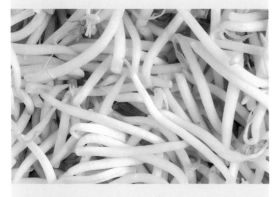

- Yeast extract
- Lentils
- Dried fruit

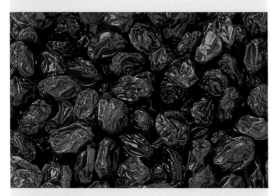

- Molasses
- Sesame seeds
- Green leafy vegetables

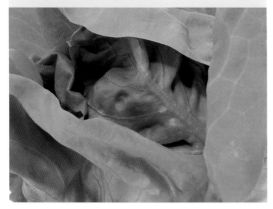

## Top sources of B12

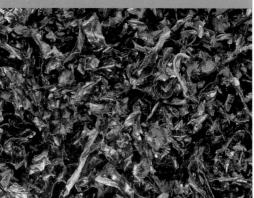

- Miso
- Tempe
- Alfalfa sprouts
- Tamari

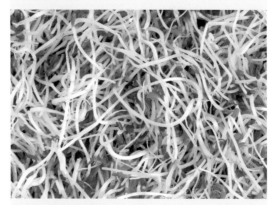

- Yeast extract
- Blue-green algae (spirulina, chlorella) and seaweeds
- Eggs (for vegetarians)
- Dairy (for vegetarians)

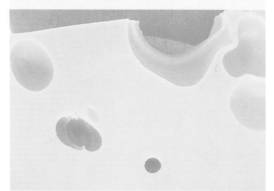

## The benefits of vegetarian and vegan diets

The benefits of following a healthy balanced vegetarian or vegan diet are endless.

### Healthy bowels

Vegetarian and vegan diets are generally much higher in both soluble and insoluble fibre, which are fundamentally important for a healthy digestive tract. Trillions of friendly bacteria colonize the small and large intestine, and these beneficial micro-organisms flourish on a high-fibre diet. As the bacteria grow they produce nourishment for the cells of the intestinal lining. They also aid with the detoxification of hormones, toxins and cholesterol, and most importantly of all they help to protect the bowel lining from bowel cancer.

### Happy hearts

There is no doubt that vegetarian and vegan diets contain less saturated fat and cholesterol than a diet that includes meat. High levels of fat and cholesterol can increase the risk of furred-up arteries and thick, sticky blood, both of which contribute to heart disease. As vegetarian and vegan diets are also high in fibre (which helps to reduce cholesterol), high in antioxidants (which strengthen artery walls) and high in vitamin E (which prevents blood fats from becoming too thick and sticky), they generally provide increased protection against cardiovascular disease.

### Acid–alkaline balance

The human body is very sensitive and many of the everyday biochemical processes occur more efficiently if the body is in an alkaline state. The food you choose to eat has a profound effect on what's known as the acid–alkaline balance. Animal and dairy products along with caffeine, alcohol, sugar and nicotine can have an acidifying effect on body fluids and tissue. Nature has, of course, cleverly balanced this out making plant-based foods, as opposed to animal-sourced foods, have an alkalising effect.

We have both noticed that some opportunistic degenerative diseases can start to take root when the body becomes too acidic for extended periods. Vegetarians, and in particular vegans, are more likely to have a better acid–alkaline balance and increased protection against degenerative diseases than meat-eaters. It is possible to supplement the diet with nutrients to help establish a more alkaline environment, but as always, it's best to do so under the supervision of a nutrition consultant.

### Strong immunity – think colour

It's not just the acid–alkaline balance that enhances your protection against illness. The increased levels of fresh fruit and vegetables in vegetarian and vegan diets bring in a rich supply of antioxidants and phytonutrients, and these plant chemicals have a good reputation for boosting body immunity. Orange and red fruits and vegetables are rich in beta-carotene and lycopene, whilst green leafy vegetables are rich in vitamin C and beta-carotene. Purple, blue and red fruits and berries are rich in pro-anthocyanadins and bioflavanols; nuts and seeds are rich in vitamin E, zinc and selenium. All these nutrients help to boost immunity and fight infections.

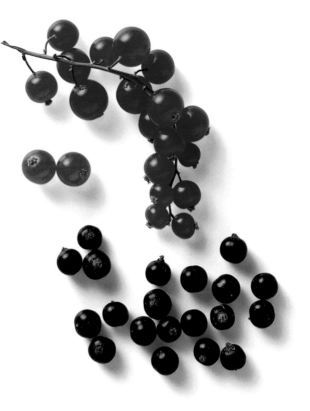

### Squeaky clean

Unfortunately, due to developments in both intensive agriculture and food processing, many of our food groups have been acted upon by chemicals that can exert a negative impact on human health. The main food groups to be affected include meat, poultry and dairy produce, as these foods often contain residues of substances such as growth promoters, antibiotics and artificial preservatives and additives.

The effects that some of these chemicals have on health is still largely unknown. Eating organic meat and dairy produce does reduce this toxic load, but abstaining completely from these food groups results in a cleaner existence.

Vegetarians and vegans do not totally avoid food toxicity since contamination also applies to the plant world. Some fruits, vegetables, pulses (legumes) and wholegrains also contain chemical residues from artificial fertilizers, fungicides and insecticides. Buying organic produce and washing or peeling fresh fruit and vegetables helps to reduce your intake of these agro-chemical food residues. It's also best to wash produce in a mixture of water and a tablespoon of vinegar as many additives are fat-based.

### Enzymes that spring clean

Both a vegetarian and vegan diet naturally involve eating high levels of fresh fruit and vegetables, which are themselves packed full of natural enzymes. These enzymes have two major health benefits – firstly, they have a direct effect on your digestion by enhancing the breakdown of foods; secondly, they are capable of being absorbed into the body where they effectively encourage the excretion of dead cells and debris from the blood and lymph, giving your body a spring clean.

## Complications of vegetarian and vegan diets

### Low on oil?

Vegetarians and vegans are at risk of having a low intake of essential fatty acids. Omega-3 oils found in oily fish are vital for a healthy brain and nervous system function and are also required during pregnancy and throughout breastfeeding. They are needed for cardiovascular protection, hormone production and promoting healthy hair, skin and nails.

The main vegetarian and vegan source of omega-3 essential fatty acids are flax oil and blue-green algae, so to prevent an omega-3 fatty acid deficiency it is important that both vegetarians and vegans include flax oil in their daily diet – preferably oil that has not been subjected to heat or light.

Flax oil is ideal drizzled over brown rice, baked potatoes or incorporated into a salad dressing. Supplementing your diet with spirulina or chlorella, available from health food shops, can further top up your omega-3 levels.

### Poor protein power

Unless careful attention is paid to protein combining in daily meal planning and cooking for both vegetarian and vegan diets, it is very easy to become protein deficient. Protein is an important component of bones, muscles, connective tissue, organs, hair, skin and nails. Proteins are also utilized to generate enzymes, hormones, immune cells and chemical messengers that influence biochemical reactions and body processes. Protein deficiency can be expressed in many different forms including weak muscles, poor bone strength, poor hair, skin and nail condition, frequent infections and poor immunity.

Amino acids are also strongly involved in brain chemistry as they are used to form the brain chemicals dopamine, adrenalin, noradrenalin

### Are you low on oil?

- Do you have dry skin, eczema or dermatitis?
- Do your eyes feel sore or gritty?
- Do you find it hard to concentrate?
- Is your memory worse than it used to be?
- Is your hair dry and frizzy?
- Do you suffer from pain and inflammation?
- Are your nails dry, weak and flaky?

If you answer yes to more than three of these questions then you may need to increase your intake of omega-3 oils.

and serotonin. These neurotransmitters are responsible for generating your feelings, emotions, mood and sleep. Poor dietary intake of amino acids, such as tryptophan, leads to imbalances between neurotransmitters. Symptoms include anxiety, nervousness, depression, paranoia, mania and insomnia. It is often this lack of amino acids that is involved in the progression of some eating disorders, as a low intake of food can exacerbate body dysmorphia and anxiety over food intake.

**A word about dairy**

As a vegetarian it is very easy to develop an overreliance on dairy produce such as cheese and yoghurt as your main source of protein. However, we believe that variety in the diet is of paramount importance.

Remember to get your protein from all food groups, whilst rotating your dairy intake. You can choose from cow's, sheep's or goat's milk products or perhaps soya instead. However, there seems to be a perception that all soya products are healthy, and whilst they do make a good protein choice, many soya products, especially yoghurts, are all too often packed with sugar and flavourings which do not match the healthy aura that soya products have. This may have more significance for vegans who will obviously be avoiding all animal products and thus perhaps more reliant on soya products. Take a look at the list of ingredients for some of the regular dairy alternatives, and you will see that some are far better for you than others.

There are many benefits to be gained by choosing to follow a vegetarian or vegan diet, but it does require not only commitment but also education and variety. It is all too easy to have a limited diet, which could mean that you are not exposed to the whole range of nutrients. We encourage you to ensure that your diet is as varied as possible – take a look at our list of 100 top foods (see pages 12–25) and see how many new foods you could include in your diet.

# vitamins, minerals and phytonutrients

| Vitamins | | | |
|---|---|---|---|
| | **What does this nutrient do?** | **Nutrient-rich foods include:** | **Deficiency signs include:** |
| **Vitamin A – Retinol and Beta-carotene** | Vitamin A is important for overall eye health and vision. This nutrient is involved in maintaining healthy skin and protects against infection, especially along mucus membranes, such as those in the nose, throat, lungs, bladder and vagina. Vitamin A is an active antioxidant, reducing toxicity and cellular damage. Beta-carotene, present in plant foods, is converted into vitamin A. | Retinol – fish liver oils, liver, butter, cheese, eggs and fortified margarines. Beta-carotene – apricots, mangoes, papaya, carrots, sweet potatoes, squash, red peppers, yellow peppers, tomatoes and green leafy vegetables. | Poor night vision, frequent colds, lung infections, thrush and cystitis. Mouth and stomach ulcers. Poor skin condition, liver spots and dry, itchy eyes. |
| **B1 – Thiamine** | Like most B-vitamins, thiamine is needed for the cellular process that converts glucose into energy. | Yeast extract, beef, organ meats, peas, pulses (legumes), brown rice, wheatgerm, soya beans, bean sprouts, nuts, avocados, cauliflower and spinach. | Fatigue, stomach pains, indigestion, constipation, depression, confusion, irritability and insomnia. |
| **B2 – Riboflavin** | Riboflavin is required as a co-factor in the formation of energy units called ATP. This nutrient is also used for proteins and fatty acid metabolism and used during the repair of mucus membranes. It is an essential nutrient for healthy hair, skin and nails. | Yeast extract, eggs, milk, liver, brown rice, mushrooms, asparagus, broccoli, avocados, Brussel sprouts, salmon, tuna, wheatgerm and nuts. | Cracks or sores in the corners of the mouth, bloodshot eyes, sensitivity to light, sore tongue, poor skin and hair condition, fatigue, depression and insomnia. |
| **B3 – Niacin** | Niacin is known to be active in more than 50 different metabolic reactions, many of which convert fats, proteins and carbohydrates into energy. Niacin is needed for the production of brain chemicals, such as serotonin, which is responsible for good moods and a sense of wellbeing. This B-vitamin is also important for cardiovascular health and protection against inflammation, and helps regulate blood glucose. | Yeast extract, chicken, turkey, beef, milk, eggs, peanuts, bean sprouts and wheatgerm. | Poor mental health including dementia, depression, anxiety, irritability and mood swings. Elevated blood pressure, cholesterol and blood triglycerides. Poor skin, hair and nail condition. Inflammatory conditions such as arthritis. |
| **B5 – Pantothenic Acid** | Pantothenic acid is utilized during the conversion of carbohydrates into energy. During times of exposure to stress, this vitamin is needed for adrenal support and formation of steroid or stress hormones. The many other roles of vitamin B5 include formation of antibodies, nervous system health and healthy hair, skin and nails. | Wholegrains, wheatgerm, kidney, liver, green vegetables, nuts, chicken and molasses. | Poor ability to cope with stress. Headaches, fatigue, restless or itchy legs and burning feet, tingling in the arms and legs. |

| | What does this nutrient do? | Nutrient-rich foods include: | Deficiency signs include: |
|---|---|---|---|
| **B6 – Pyridoxine** | Vitamin B6 has long been associated with female health issues due to its involvement with oestrogen metabolism and hormone balance. It is also involved in the production of brain chemicals required to maintain blood sugar levels, nervous system health and formation of red blood cells. Also helps to prevent homocysteine levels from becoming too excessive. | Yeast extract, chicken, beef, lamb, fish, egg yolks, soya beans, bananas, avocados, cabbage, cauliflower, prunes, walnuts, pulses (legumes) and brown rice. | Depression, mental confusion, PMS, fertility problems, mood swings, irritability, tingling hands and feet and poor dream recall. |
| **B12 – Cyanoco-balamin** | This is essential for the formation of healthy red blood cells. It also protects against homocysteine levels which are associated with heart disease. B12 is required for the insulation of nerve fibres. | Liver, kidney, clams, oysters, crab, salmon, sardines, egg yolks, lobster, scallops, swordfish, tuna, fermented soya beans (tempe, tamari) and chicken. | Pernicious anaemia, dizziness, pallor, numbness, tingling, sore tongue, period pains, brain fatigue and nerve degeneration. |
| **Biotin** | Biotin is used to convert fats, carbohydrates and proteins into energy. It is also needed for healthy hair and skin, for nervous system function and for the production of brain chemicals. Biotin is involved in folic acid metabolism as it converts this nutrient into its active form. | Brown rice, nuts, fruit, egg yolks, liver and kidney. | Depression, fatigue, poor appetite, hair loss, premature greying hair and dry skin. |
| **Vitamin C** | This nutrient has powerful antioxidant properties and protects both cells and the constituents of the blood from free-radical damage. Vitamin C helps to restore and regenerate the antioxidant potential of vitamin E. As an important nutrient for collagen formation vitamin C helps to build strong flexible arteries, capillaries, bones, skin, hair, nails, teeth, cartilage, tendons and scar tissue. It helps combat the effects of stress as it is utilized for the synthesis and release of stress hormones. Vitamin C influences mood as it is required for the synthesis of brain chemicals, such as serotonin. Iron absorption is greatly increased by the presence of vitamin C within the intestine. Vitamin C largely influences immunity by stimulating immune cells to fight infections and through chelating heavy metals from the body. It also protects the cardiovascular system by influencing cholesterol excretion. | Lemons, limes, oranges, tangerines, grapefruit, blackcurrants, gooseberries, guava, kiwi fruit, lychees, papaya, raspberries, parsley, spinach, green beans, peas, broccoli, Brussels sprouts, cabbage, cauliflower, kale, peppers, spring greens and watercress. | Frequent colds and infections, poor skin, hair and nail tone, poor wound healing and bleeding gums. |

| | What does this nutrient do? | Nutrient rich foods include: | Deficiency signs include: |
|---|---|---|---|
| **Vitamin D – Cholecalciferol** | This nutrient's primary role is that of calcium metabolism. Vitamin D is responsible for increasing intestinal absorption of calcium and phosphorous whilst increasing the deposition of calcium into bones. | Oily fish, liver, egg yolks, cheese, milk and fortified margarines. The body manufactures vitamin D in skin that is exposed to sunlight. | Poor bone strength and poor bone formation (particularly in children), tooth decay, muscle weakness and muscle spasms. |
| **Vitamin E – Tocopherols** | A powerful antioxidant that works closely with vitamin C and selenium to protect body cells against harmful effects of free-radical damage and toxins. Vitamin E provides protection to the cardiovascular system by preventing blood lipids from becoming oxidized and sticky. This nutrient also protects body tissues from premature ageing and has anti-cancer properties. Vitamin E is strongly associated with reproductive health and fertility. | Wheatgerm, safflower oil, avocados, almonds, peanuts, walnuts, sunflower seeds, sesame seeds, pecans, cashew nuts, sweet potatoes, tuna, olive oil, eggs, butter and green leafy vegetables. | High blood pressure, atherosclerosis, thrombosis, poor skin tone and fertility problems. |
| **Folic acid** | Folic acid is the third and final vitamin to protect the body from excessive homocysteine levels. Required for red blood cell formation and maintaining a healthy nervous system, it is utilized in the formation of brain chemicals that control sleep and pain and regulate mood. Especially important during pregnancy due to its effects on protein synthesis and for the prevention of spina bifida. | Green leafy vegetables, kidney beans, broccoli, beets, cauliflower, peas, green beans, sweet potatoes, asparagus, brown rice and lima beans. | Anaemia, fatigue, breathlessness, depression, irritability, confusion and insomnia. |
| **Vitamin K – Phylloquinone** | This vitamin is important for the formation of prothrombin, a blood constituent responsible for producing clotting at the site of a wound or cut. | Cabbage, kale, spinach, parsley, broccoli, yoghurt, kelp, oily fish and potatoes. A considerable quantity of highly absorbable vitamin K is manufactured by good bacteria living within the intestine. | Poor wound healing, poor blood clotting, nose bleeds and easy bruising. |

## Minerals

| | What does this nutrient do? | Nutrient-rich foods include: | Deficiency signs include: |
|---|---|---|---|
| **Boron** | Boron has a large role to play in carbohydrate, fat and calcium metabolism. This mineral also helps to reduce inflammation, protect connective tissue and influence bone density. | Water, legumes and most fruits and vegetables. | Poor bone density and difficulty with weight loss. |
| **Calcium** | Calcium provides structure and strength to the skeletal system. Calcium has a large role to play in nerve impulse transmission and muscle contraction. This mineral is also involved in blood clotting and maintaining normal blood pressure. | Spring greens, spinach, okra, kale, broccoli, tofu, sardines, whitebait, anchovies, pilchards, yoghurt, cottage cheese, almonds, hazelnuts, sunflower seeds, sesame seeds and peas. | Poor bone density, tooth decay, muscle cramps or spasms, constipation or diarrhoea and twitches. |

| | What does this nutrient do? | Nutrient-rich foods include: | Deficiency signs include: |
|---|---|---|---|
| **Chromium** | Chromium is a component of 'glucose tolerance factor', which influences blood sugar balance through insulin metabolism. Chromium is also linked to the cardiovascular system since it has a positive influence on cholesterol levels. | Egg yolks, molasses, liver, kidney, wholegrains, nuts, mushrooms and asparagus. | Irritability, sugar cravings, mood swings, thirst, sweating, tingling legs and arms, dizziness and energy dips. |
| **Iodine** | Iodine is the main component of the hormone thyroxin. This hormone influences our metabolic rate, in other words the speed at which all body processes occur. | Seaweeds, kelp, seafood and garlic. | Weight gain, constipation, low energy, sensitivity to the cold, cold hands and feet and dry skin. |
| **Iron** | Iron is the major component of red blood cell haemoglobin. Haemoglobin picks up, transports and delivers oxygen to every cell in the body. Without oxygen, body cells are unable to 'breathe', generate energy or carry out their daily functions. Iron is also important for optimum immunity. | Spinach, spring greens, kale, lentils, whitebait, sardines, prawns, liver, kidney, venison, oatcakes, rye bread, wheatgerm, quinoa, watercress, sesame seeds and cashew nuts. | Anaemia, pallor, low energy and breathlessness. |
| **Magnesium** | Magnesium is required for many of the enzyme systems involved in converting fats, proteins and carbohydrates into energy. This mineral stimulates muscles to relax and works with calcium to activate nerve transmission. Magnesium is crucial for the proper functioning of heart and intestinal muscles. In the presence of magnesium, the body can deposit calcium into bones and teeth, making this an important mineral for bone density. Magnesium is considered to be one of the stress-busting nutrients since it enables the adrenal glands to produce stress hormones. This mineral has a role to play in the production of many body hormones, including sex hormones. | Spinach, kale, okra, broccoli, peas, anchovies, brown rice, quinoa, oatcakes, figs, sunflower seeds, sesame seeds, almonds, Brazil nuts, prawns and lentils. | Muscle cramps, inability to cope with stress, heart palpitations, constipation, insomnia, anxiety, poor bone density, tooth decay and high blood pressure. |
| **Manganese** | This nutrient is a co-factor in over 20 enzyme systems which influence growth and tissue repair, nervous system function, energy production, blood sugar control, female hormone production, thyroxin production and bone density. Manganese is vital for cellular protection and detoxification because it activates the antioxidant system, superoxide dismutase (SOD). This mineral is also strongly linked with the protection and formation of synovial fluid in joint spaces. | Quorn, green and brown lentils, rye bread, wheatgerm, brown rice, oatmeal, quinoa, buckwheat, pine nuts, pecans, walnuts, sesame seeds, hazelnuts, pineapple and macadamia nuts. | Poor blood sugar control, reduced fertility and joint pains. |

| | What does this nutrient do? | Nutrient-rich foods include: | Deficiency signs include: |
|---|---|---|---|
| **Molybdenum** | Molybdenum helps the body to utilize iron. It is also important for heavy metal and petrochemical detoxification. | Pork, lamb, lentils, beans and tomatoes. | Tooth decay, joint pains and an increased susceptibility to the effects of pollution. |
| **Phosphorous** | Every cell in the body has a phospholipid membrane composed of phosphorous, fat and protein. So this mineral is a vital component of every body cell and tissue. The brain and nervous system are highly concentrated with phospholipid membranes, making this a vital nutrient for brain and nervous system health. Phosphorous is used to activate B-vitamins and works with calcium and magnesium to maintain strong bone density. | Watercress, quorn, garlic, Brussels sprouts, sesame seeds, almonds, Brazil nuts and cashew nuts. | Weakness, joint stiffness and fragile bones. |
| **Potassium** | Potassium is an important body electrolyte, helping to control correct water balance. It stimulates muscular contractions and nerve transmission. Potassium is required by body cells in order to respond to thyroxin, the hormone that controls our metabolic rate. | Watercress, potatoes, kiwi fruit, figs, bananas, avocados, spring greens, spinach, sweet potatoes, parsnips, onions, radishes, garlic, celery, cauliflower, bean sprouts, courgettes, broccoli, lentils, pine nuts, pistachios, almonds, hazelnuts, peanuts, asparagus, scallops and millet. | Pins and needles, muscle weakness, low blood pressure, thirst, cellulite, palpitations and constipation. |
| **Selenium** | Selenium has a reputation for being highly protective against cancer. This mineral is an important co-factor in the body's enzyme detoxification system and acts as a powerful antioxidant. Selenium protects against heavy metal toxicity. | Mushrooms, kidney beans, green and brown lentils, houmous, black-eye beans, prawns, lobster, crab, tuna, trout, swordfish, sardines, herrings, mackerel, sole, plaice, cod, kidney, brown rice, liver, onions, Brazil nuts, sesame seeds, sunflower seeds and cashew nuts. | Increased risk of cancer, poor immune function and signs of premature ageing. |
| **Sulphur** | Sulphur gives stability and strength to protein structures by acting as a bridge, linking strands of proteins together in the formation of body cells and tissue. This mineral is important for healthy hair, skin, nails and bones. Sulphur is also important for liver detoxification and anti-inflammatory reactions. | Fish, eggs, cabbage, onions and garlic. | Poor hair, skin and nail health. |
| **Zinc** | Zinc is involved in insulin storage and activity, making this mineral important for blood sugar control. Zinc is also a vital nutrient for immunity since it is required for the formation and activation of T-cells and helps the body fight viruses. Also important for skin tone and cell growth and repair. Plays a role in sex hormone production. | Quorn, peas, tofu, chickpeas, mussels, crab, prawns, lobster, squid, sardines, anchovies, liver, kidney, chicken, turkey, oatcakes, oats, brown rice, wheatgerm, quinoa, buckwheat noodles, lean lamb, lean beef, pine nuts, cashew nuts and pumpkin seeds. | Frequent infections, poor skin tone, irritability, mood swings, energy dips, fertility problems, PMS and poor wound healing. |

## Phytonutrients

| | What does this nutrient do? | Nutrient-rich foods include: | Deficiency signs include: |
|---|---|---|---|
| **Bioflavanols** | These special plant chemicals act as powerful antioxidants, neutralizing free radicals and harmful toxins, protecting cells from damage. They strengthen capillary walls and prevent blood from becoming too sticky, making them great for cardiovascular health. Bioflavanols also help vitamin C to work efficiently and effectively within the body. | Citrus fruits, purple and red berries and highly coloured vegetables. | Frequent infections such as colds and flu, thread veins or varicose veins and a generally poor immune system. |
| **Phyto-oestrogen** | These plant chemicals have a similar structure to oestrogen. It is this structural similarity that allows these phyto-oestrogens to fit into cellular receptor sites and exert an oestrogen effect on body cells. Phyto-oestrogens are considered to be oestrogen modulators. When natural oestrogens are too low, they sit in receptor sites and top up the oestrogen activity needed. However, when exposure to powerful synthetic oestrogens has been too high, phyto-oestrogens in the receptor sites block the activity of synthetic oestrogens and dampen down the natural oestrogenic activity within the body. | Fennel, soya milk, tofu, tempe, tamari, flax seeds, oats, celery, alfalfa and rhubarb. | PMS, endometriosis, polycystic ovaries, menopause, osteoporosis and prostate cancer. |
| **Plant sterols** | Plant sterols support adrenal function, helping to combat the effects of prolonged exposure to stress, support immune function, protect the cardiovascular system and calm inflammation. | Nuts, seeds, pulses (legumes) and mushrooms. | Ongoing immune problems, frequent infections, asthma, arthritis and eczema. |

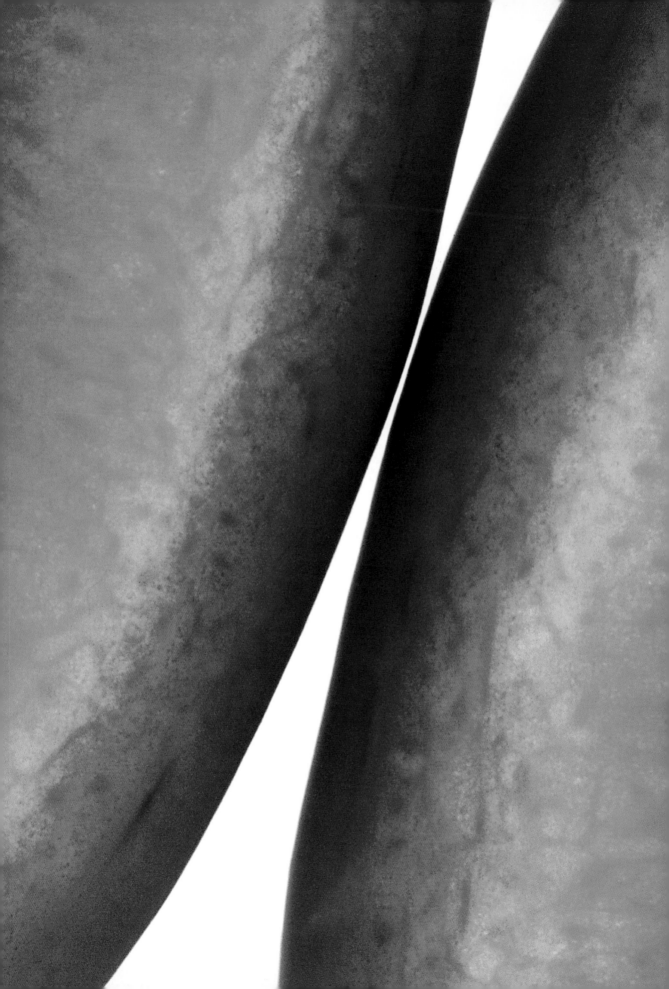

# part one

# Energy and Emotions

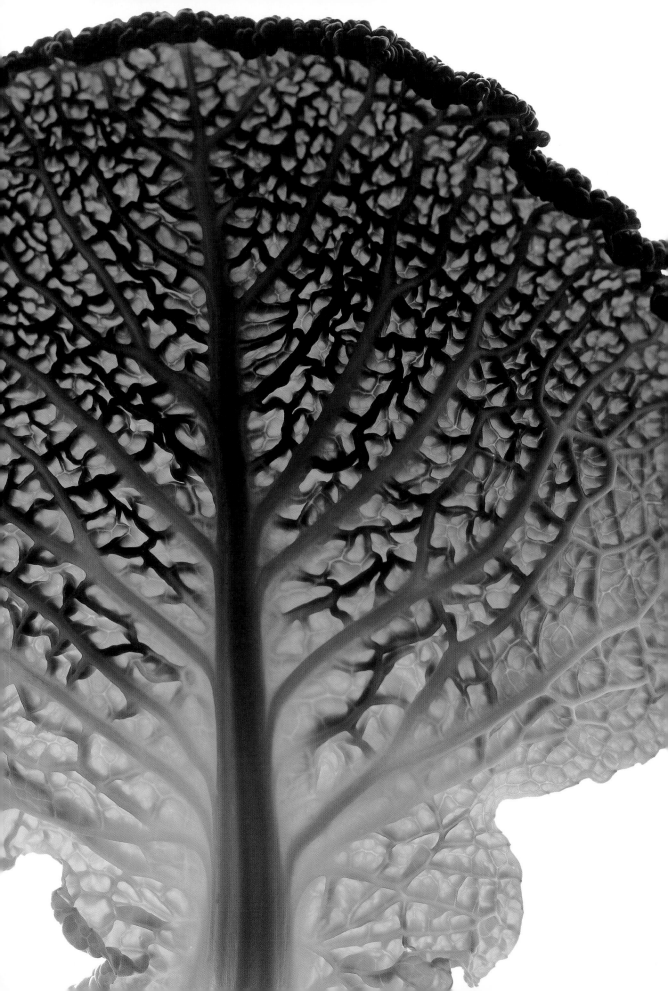

# good food, good mood

The food we eat is used to make the energy required for every function in the body – from walking and talking to digesting and breathing. But why do we often complain of a lack of energy, or of feeling irritable and listless? The answer lies in the type of foods that make up our daily diet.

## Energy boosting

As well as water and air, we require a constant, regular intake of food to provide the major source of energy for movement, breathing, heat regulation, heart function, blood circulation and brainpower. It is staggering to realize that, even at rest, our brain uses approximately 50 per cent of the energy that is derived from the food we consume, and considerably more than that when we actively engage our minds, such as in a period of intense work or when sitting an exam. So how is the food transformed into energy?

The process of digestion, described more fully in the digestion section (see pages 84–95), breaks down all carbohydrates into single molecules of glucose, which are then transported through the gut wall into the bloodstream. This glucose is carried to the liver, where it is filtered and stored ready for use. The pituitary gland in the brain directs a series of hormonal releases from the pancreas and adrenal gland, which stimulate the liver to release the stores of glucose back into the bloodstream to be delivered to whichever cells, organs and muscles require it.

Once it reaches its target organ, the glucose enters individual cells where it is converted into units of energy called ATP, which the cells use. The process of keeping the organs supplied with energy is known as blood sugar management.

To maximize our energy, we need to include certain foods in our diets, especially those that boost the metabolism and those that sustain consistent energy levels. To understand how these foods benefit us, we need to consider the following factors.

### How does food become energy?

Every cell contains several mitochondria. Here, the constituent parts of food undergo a series of chemical reactions, producing energy as ATP. In this way, each cell acts like a tiny power plant. It is interesting to note that the number of mitochondria we have in each of our cells is dependent upon our energy needs. If we exercise regularly, the number of mitochondria increases to meet the demand for higher energy production. Conversely, leading a sedentary lifestyle will lead to a decrease of energy output

LEFT Cabbage contains the minerals required for concentration and good moods.

efficiency, and a correspondingly lower number of mitochondria. These chemical reactions require the presence of a large number of nutrients (B-vitamins, vitamin C and magnesium), each of which is specific to different parts of the process of energy production (see Energy foods, page 61). Apart from the importance of an individual food's nutrient content, it is also vital to eat certain types of food. In order to obtain sustained energy, a balance of complex carbohydrates, essential fatty acids and proteins needs to be eaten.

It is important to keep blood glucose at an even level for concentration and alertness (see Blood

and the muscles. It is stored in the form of glycogen, which is easily converted back into glucose when required. During the 'fight or flight' response (see page 59), glycogen is released into the bloodstream to make extra energy available for the body.

### Protein balanced with carbohydrates

While everyone's diet should contain a mix of carbohydrates and protein, each individual has a personal level at which the two are optimally balanced, depending on lifestyle. Achieving your personal balance can only be done through trial and error, but the quantities on the table opposite provide a guideline.

## It is important to minimize those dietary factors that rob the body of energy or interfere with energy production. All such foods stimulate the hormone adrenaline.

sugar management, pages 60–64). Eating foods that have a low glycaemic value will help to maintain blood sugar levels. Adding some protein and fibre to every meal or snack will help to sustain consistent energy levels throughout the day.

### Carbohydrates and glucose

The energy that we derive from food is more likely to come from carbohydrates than from protein or fat. Carbohydrates are more easily converted into energy, and are therefore the most convenient food for the body to use to manufacture energy.

Glucose can be turned into immediate energy, and any excess is kept as a reserve in the liver

Take care with your protein intake. Always match your protein intake with high-quality complex carbohydrates such as dense vegetables or wholegrains. Eating too much protein shifts the body into an acid state, while it should be slightly alkaline. The body's built-in buffering systems work to change an acid state to an alkaline one by releasing calcium from the bones. Eventually this can compromise bone health, leading to the bone-thinning disease osteoporosis, in which fractures readily occur.

Experiment by increasing your protein intake a little and decreasing your carbohydrates, or vice versa, until you feel your energy levels are higher and remain consistent.

| Your lifestyle | What you need (ratio of protein to carbohydrate) |
| --- | --- |
| **INACTIVE** Elderly, sedentary, recuperating | **protein 1 : 2 carbohydrate** |
| **MORE ACTIVE** Office worker, shopkeeper, homemaker | **protein 1 : 1$\frac{1}{2}$ carbohydrate** |
| **ACTIVE LIFESTYLE** Exercising regularly, working mother, student | **protein 1 : 1$\frac{1}{4}$ carbohydrate** |
| **MOST ACTIVE** Athlete or bodybuilder, ballerina | **protein 1 : 1 carbohydrate** |

## Energy requirements during life

At various times during our lives we need extra energy. For example, in childhood we need energy for growth and learning, while during adolescence it is required for the hormonal and physical changes that take place in the body. During pregnancy, both mother and baby place extra demands on energy supplies, and throughout our lives we use up extra energy during periods of stress. In addition, if you have an active life and/or a non-sedentary job, you will need more energy than those who do not.

## Energy stealers

It is important to minimize those dietary factors that rob the body of energy or interfere with energy production. These include alcohol, tea, coffee and fizzy drinks, as well as cakes, biscuits and sweets. All such foods stimulate the hormone adrenaline, which is made by the adrenal glands. Adrenaline is produced primarily when the body perceives a threat or a challenge – the 'fight or flight' syndrome – to prepare itself for action. It causes the heart to beat faster, the lungs to take in more air, the liver to release extra glucose into the blood, and blood to divert from non-vital areas to where it will be of more use, such as the legs. If adrenaline is constantly over-produced because of stimulant foods or emotional stress, it may lead to general fatigue.

Stress is also an energy stealer, because it encourages the release of stored glucose from the liver and muscles, providing short-term energy but long-term fatigue, as energy stores are constantly being depleted. During the 'fight or flight' response, the liver releases glycogen (stored sugars) into the blood, raising blood sugar. Therefore prolonged exposure to stress can play havoc with blood sugar levels. In the same way, caffeine and stimulants such as nicotine in cigarettes also raise blood sugar by stressing the adrenal glands – these release two hormones, cortisol and adrenaline, which interfere with the digestive process and direct the liver to release stored glycogen.

### Energy foods

The most important energy foods are those rich in the B-complex group of vitamins, which comprises vitamins B1, B2, B3, B5, B6, B12, B9 (folic acid) and biotin. They are all found in abundance in the wholegrains of millet, brown rice, buckwheat, rye, quinoa (a South American grain that is becoming more widely available), corn and barley. If these grains are sprouted, their energy quotient is increased many times, as the enzyme action involved in the sprouting process increases the nutrient value. The range of B-complex vitamins is also to be found in fresh green vegetables.

Other nutrients that are required for energy production are vitamin C, found in fruit and vegetables such as oranges, potatoes and peppers; magnesium, which is found in green vegetables, nuts and seeds; zinc, from egg yolks, fish and sunflower seeds; iron, plentiful in grains, pumpkin seeds and lentils; copper, part of the make-up of Brazil nuts, oats, salmon and mushrooms; and co-enzyme Q10, found in beef, sardines, spinach and peanuts.

## Blood sugar management

How many times have you woken up feeling groggy, bad-tempered and in need of another couple of hours' sleep? You don't feel equipped to start the day. Or perhaps, having reached mid-morning, you wonder how you will manage to continue until your lunch break.

Worse still, how often do you feel exhausted by mid-afternoon, knowing that you have several more hours of work to do, the journey home to cope with, and then dinner to cook and eat? Do you ask yourself, 'Whatever happened to all that energy I used to have?'

Constant fatigue and lack of energy can have many different causes but, quite often, they are the result of a poor and/or irregular diet, and the increasing consumption of stimulants to 'keep going' throughout the day. Depression, irritability and mood swings, as well as premenstrual tension and outbursts of anger, anxiety and nervousness can all be the result of imbalances in energy production, nutrient deficiencies and frequent fad dieting.

Understanding the basics of energy production in the body shows us how we can, within a remarkably short time, ensure a higher and more constant level of energy all day long – and still have enough stamina to enjoy the latter part of the day, as well as experiencing more restorative sleep during the night.

### Simple and complex sugars

The sugar present in food is in the form of complex sugars. The body has a lot of work to do to break these complex sugars down into the simplest sugar unit, glucose. This conversion process has the effect of slowly releasing glucose into the bloodstream in a manageable fashion.

Your body keeps around one teaspoon of glucose in the bloodstream at any one time. If your blood sugar falls below or above this level then symptoms such as irritability, mood

# Energy foods – as simple as ABC

**There are three different grades of energy food – A, B and C. The A-grade foods are the most effective. The B-grade foods also provide good levels of energy, but not quite as much as the A-foods. C-grade foods provide 'cheap' energy – you get a quick energy surge, but it is not lasting. At times when extra energy is required, try to eat lots of small meals throughout the day that include A- or B-grade carbohydrates and protein.**

## A-grade foods

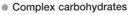

- **Complex carbohydrates**
  Wholegrains such as oats, barley, brown rice, millet, wholegrain bread, rye bread, corn bread
- **Vegetables**
  Dense vegetables such as broccoli, cauliflower, Brussels sprouts, mushrooms, turnips, carrots (especially raw), asparagus, artichokes, spinach
- **Fruit**
  Avocados, apples, pears, pineapples, berries – strawberries, raspberries, blackberries, cherries
- **Protein**
  Fish including salmon, tuna, herring and mackerel, seaweeds, eggs, tofu, walnuts, Brazil nuts, sunflower seeds, pumpkin seeds, sesame seeds, linseeds, sprouted seeds and grains, haricot and lima beans, chickpeas, lentils, soya beans

## B-grade foods

- **Complex carbohydrates**
  Buckwheat, red macrobiotic rice, wild rice, oatcakes
- **Vegetables**
  Potatoes, sweet potatoes, corn, squashes, beetroot, peppers, wild rice, yam, watercress, salad leaves
- **Fruit**
  Peaches, apricots, mangoes, papayas, bananas
- **Protein**
  Kidney beans, black beans, peas (dried/split), almonds, chicken, game, turkey, venison, nut butters, yoghurt, cottage cheese

## C-grade foods

- **Processed carbohydrates**
  White pasta, bread, white rice, rice noodles, egg noodles
- **Vegetables**
  Green peas, courgettes (zucchini), cucumbers
- **Fruit**
  Tomatoes, prunes, all dried fruit, grapes, figs
- **Protein**
  Dairy products such as cheese and milk, beef, lamb, veal

61

swings, sugar cravings, thirst, headaches, energy dips and dizziness may be experienced. A diet too high in carbohydrates can cause blood sugar levels to fluctuate – balancing carbohydrates with fibre and protein helps to reduce this.

When food is digested and absorbed into the bloodstream, hormones trigger the pancreas to release insulin to help transport glucose across the individual cell membranes. If the level of sugar (glucose) in the bloodstream is in excess of what the body requires, the surplus is sent to the liver to be stored until needed.

Most commercial foods, fast foods, cereals (granolas), cakes, confectionery, biscuits and soft drinks are loaded with simple sugars, which rush into the bloodstream increasing blood sugar levels too rapidly. The pancreas responds by releasing a large dose of insulin. This insulin can effectively transport too much of the glucose out of the blood into the cells, leaving blood sugar levels too low. This results in the highs and lows that many people experience after eating a sweet snack. A bar of chocolate may be a great 'pick-me-up', giving a quick fix of energy, but within a short space of time the eater will feel more lethargic than he or she did to start with. This pancreatic reaction is known as reactive hypoglycaemia.

### nutrition know-how

Drinking tea or coffee for a quick boost creates unnecessary stress on the body and provides only short-lived energy. Replace with green tea, which is low in caffeine and high in antioxidant action, or diluted orange juice.

Over an extended period, it can lead to maturity-onset diabetes, unless changes are made to the diet. The production and release of insulin from the pancreas is initiated by vitamin B3 (niacin) and the mineral chromium, which work together. Chromium is frequently found to be deficient in those who suffer from reactive hypoglycaemia and those with poor diets, as the pancreas becomes overworked and exhausted.

### Insulin facts

Both insulin and glucose are highly oxidizing, which means they are capable of damaging body cells and tissues. When insulin and glucose reach excessive levels in the blood, damage to blood cells, eye tissue, kidney tissue and synovial fluid can occur. Excessive levels of insulin have also been linked to conditions such as obesity, heart disease and polycystic ovarian syndrome.

### Insidious sugar

Sugar is the greatest disturber of the body's energy production processes. And sugar is insidious. It is not only found in obvious foods such as sweets, cakes and canned drinks, but it is also hidden in many other items such as ready meals, prepared sauces, most cereals (granolas), bread and pizzas. Sugar is everywhere.

To see how much sugar is in a food or drink that you consume regularly, take a look at the label. The ingredients are listed in order of quantity. On a bar of chocolate, you may well discover that sugar is its most abundant ingredient, while cocoa is much further down the list, begging the question, is it a chocolate bar or a sugar bar? When you look at the label on a ready-made food item, sugar is almost always present. It is worth asking *why* sugar is included in some dishes – if you were to cook the same food at home you would not add any sugar, so why do manufacturers? The reason is quite simple: they put sugar in food because it is relatively cheap and provides a familiar and allegedly enhanced flavour – but, as nutritionists, we maintain its inclusion is unnecessary.

**Sugar in the morning, sugar in the evening**

Often we have no idea how much sugar we are eating, because it is so often present in foods we

You may also be surprised to find out how much sugar is lurking in foods we would consider to be healthy, such as yoghurt, some fruit juices, canned baked beans and other vegetables. Even the more natural forms of sugar, such as honey and molasses, will disturb your blood sugar balance. Eating such sugar-rich foods will raise your blood sugar levels, interfere with insulin release and stress your body.

Alcohol, in all forms, behaves like simple sugars as it is absorbed directly through the stomach

To become more sugar-aware, try this: avoid all sugar for two weeks. After two weeks have elapsed, try eating a spoonful of white sugar – the taste will seem overpoweringly sweet and it should turn you off sugar for quite a while.

do not expect to contain it. Look at a typical day: the Western daily breakfast of cereal (granola), toast and coffee will probably contain sugar in at least two, if not three, of the items – sugar is present in bread and cereals (granolas), and may be added to coffee. This also holds true for a typical mid-morning snack of a couple of biscuits and a canned drink. Lunch of a sandwich, a cereal (granola) bar and another canned drink will have sugar in the bread, possibly in the sandwich filling, in the cereal (granola) bar and the canned drink. Chomping through a mid-afternoon snack of biscuits, chocolate and tea piles on more sugar. Even the evening meal, perhaps pasta and a store-bought sauce, or maybe a ready-made meal, also has an extremely high sugar content.

and into the bloodstream. This is why drinking on an empty stomach can have such a rapid effect: the alcohol goes straight to the brain, affecting speech and judgement (especially when driving), and causing a loss of balance and coherence. If you are going to drink alcohol, make sure you eat something first, because this will slow down the release of alcohol into the bloodstream. However, drinking and driving, regardless of what has been eaten, is obviously dangerous and illegal.

Most fruits are digested rapidly, particularly when eaten on an empty stomach, and can have a similar effect on blood sugar balance to eating sugar, albeit to a lesser degree. Therefore people who suffer from fluctuations of energy, mood swings and fatigue would be ill-advised to follow diets where fruit is only eaten before midday. Although beneficial as antioxidants and

Some foods are known to release their sugars quickly, while others do so more slowly. It is the latter that should make up the greater part of our diets. Foods all have what is known as a

## Sugar release times

Foods release their sugars at different rates. The most beneficial are the moderate- to slow-release sugars, which provide a consistent release of sugar throughout the day. Avoid quick-release foods, which provide a sugar surge, but deplete the body's energy reserves very speedily, leaving you feeling even more tired than before.

**Quick-release sugars**
- honey
- canned drinks
- sweets and chocolate
- white rice and rice cakes
- French bread
- cornflakes
- baked potatoes
- raisins
- apricots
- cooked root vegetables

**Moderate-release sugars**
- dried fruits
- popcorn
- corn chips
- brown rice
- pasta
- bagels

**Slow-release sugars**
- rye bread
- yoghurt (unsweetened)
- pulses (legumes) includin kidney and lima beans, le and chickpeas
- wholegrains such as mill buckwheat, brown rice, quinoa
- fresh fruits, especially apples
- all raw root vegetables

a good source of fibre, fruit should be eaten in moderation when attempting to rebalance blood sugar levels – and in some cases, avoided.

### What goes up, must come down

The most effective way of keeping your blood sugar levels constant is to avoid processed sugars and to include protein in every meal. Protein encourages a series of hormonal secretions that slows down the release of sugars. Protein sources such as nuts, legumes, beans, tofu, eggs, fish and poultry are ideal. For example, after a meal of plain pasta with a tomato sauce, blood sugar will rise sharply, leading to a fall soon after. Adding some protein, such as tofu or chicken, will slow down the digestive process and help to create a more consistent blood sugar level. The protein should be combined with fibre, which slows down sugar release and makes successful blood sugar management more likely.

'glycaemic value' and the higher the value, the more quickly the sugars in the food will affect blood sugar levels. However, be aware that juicing raw vegetables, such as carrots, gives them a high glycaemic index, because the fibre content which slows digestion (and thus sugar release) has been removed. The different rates of sugar release in various foods are outlined in the box above.

## Sleeping tight – beating insomnia

Many of us experience the occasional sleepless night but, for some, this can be a regular occurrence, causing fatigue, irritability and affecting memory and concentration. Sleep is essential for body rebuilding. During the night, human growth hormone triggers proteins throughout the body to build new cells and repair any damage. It is only released when we sleep, so adequate daily (or nightly) rest is imperative to maintain a healthy body.

Stress and all stimulants, such as alcohol, tea, coffee and cola drinks, chocolate and drugs (both prescription and recreational), interfere with sound sleep patterns, as do heavy meals late in the evening, indigestion and poor blood sugar management. Dietary factors are also implicated, so if you do not sleep well, it is worth examining what you eat towards the end of the day.

Saturated fatty foods, such as dairy products, red meats and hard cheeses, all take a considerable time for the body to digest, so it is advisable to avoid these in the evening. Instead it is preferable to choose grilled fish and vegetables, rice dishes and salads, as they are less taxing for the digestive system. After dinner, herbal teas such as peppermint (aids digestion) and camomile (relaxing) are perfect alternatives to caffeinated teas and coffees.

Foods containing tyramine, an amino acid found in the nightshade family of vegetables, such as tomatoes, aubergines, courgettes (zucchini), potatoes and spinach, all stimulate the production of the hormone adrenaline, which may interfere with a good night's sleep. Tyramine is also found in alcohol, bacon, ham and sausage, so keeping these to a minimum at dinner is advisable.

## Try this simple quiz to see how well you are managing your blood sugar

If blood sugar is raised rapidly, it will come crashing down with the release of insulin, leaving you tired and craving something to get you going again. This roller-coaster of blood sugar highs and lows greatly affects our feelings and energy levels. Learning how to restore balance is one of the fundamental factors for good health.

1   Do you feel you need more than 7 hours' sleep a night?

2   Do you feel sluggish and heavy in the mornings?

3   Do you need a pick-me-up to start the day (tea, coffee, a cigarette)?

4   Do you drink tea and coffee regularly throughout the day?

5   Do you sip soft drinks (sodas) throughout the day?

6   Do you urinate frequently?

7   Do your palms sweat?

8   Do you smoke?

9   Do you look forward to an alcoholic drink in the evening?

10  Do you get very thirsty but find that the thirst is not relieved by drinking water?

11  Do you feel sleepy during the day?

12  Do you crave sugar, bread or carbohydrates through the day?

13  Do you avoid exercising, due to tiredness?

14  Do you lose concentration from time to time?

15  Do you get dizzy or irritable if you don't eat often?

If you have answered 'yes' to three or more of these questions, it is possible that you have a blood sugar management problem. Try and follow our recommendations and see if there is an improvement.

If your score is above five, then blood sugar problems are more than likely. You should follow our recommendations. If there is no improvement, you should see your doctor and/or a nutritionist for further investigation.

The specific nutrients involved in sleep problems are the minerals calcium and magnesium. Any deficiency of either can precipitate mild to severe insomnia. It is worth increasing foods that contain them to see if your sleep improves. Try including the following in your evening meal: broccoli, cauliflower, Brussels sprouts, mackerel, peas, chicken, salmon, greens and kale.

Another amino acid, tryptophan, is produced by the brain to help regulate sleep. A rich supply of it is found in bananas, turkey, tuna, figs, dates, nut butters and wholegrain crackers. Including any of these foods with dinner, or as a late-night snack, will help to promote sound sleep.

### nutrition know-how

Eating fish with green vegetables for dinner will help promote a good night's sleep, as these foods are rich in calcium and magnesium, necessary both for brain chemistry balance and to relax the body.

## PMS – the monthly monster

Not every woman suffers from premenstrual syndrome (PMS) but, for those who do, there often seems to be no escape from the monster that arrives with hideous, cyclical regularity. For some women, PMS is purely physical, causing a range of symptoms, particularly lower back pain, abdominal cramps, swollen and tender breasts and water retention. These range from being uncomfortable to extremely unpleasant.

For others, however, there are also emotional symptoms, which make PMS nothing short of a prison sentence. The symptoms can start anywhere from mid-cycle to just a few days before the onset of menstruation. For these women, irritability and mood swings, anger or violent outbursts – even thoughts of suicide – are features that the sufferer is unable to control, making her withdrawn and antisocial. These women often describe their experiences as 'having someone else move into my head', and they are frequently surprised by some of their own uncharacteristic behaviour. In many cases, it is husbands and partners who are the quickest to identify the symptoms and attribute them to their true cause.

### Hormonal balance

One of the major causes of PMS is an imbalance of the hormones oestrogen and progesterone. Although such imbalances may be 'natural', in that they occur without outside triggers, there are also many other factors that can cause PMS.

Every day we are exposed to many products (such as plastic containers and food wraps) that have oestrogen-like properties that can upset the normal levels of oestrogen circulating in the body. Oestrogen naturally drops mid-cycle, to allow progesterone levels to increase (progesterone is the hormone that supports a potential pregnancy), so an excessive amount of oestrogen will disturb this delicate balance.

Poor blood sugar management is also a contributing factor in PMS – eating a lot of sugar, simple carbohydrates and processed foods will adversely affect blood sugar levels. Also, a high sugar intake depletes the body's stores of magnesium, a primary nutrient required for muscle relaxation. Therefore, period pains and cramps can be relieved by increasing magnesium-rich foods such as wholegrains, green leafy vegetables, dairy products, fish and seafood.

B-complex vitamins are necessary for relaxation, reduction of breast tenderness and water retention, support of the adrenal glands and stress management. Wholegrains are good sources: millet, rye, buckwheat and brown rice.

### PMS and food cravings

Premenstrual food cravings are common – and they usually include stimulants such as tea, coffee and alcohol, all of which disturb blood sugar management, stress-hormone output, and consequently one's mood. Eating small meals regularly throughout the day will help to reduce cravings.

Prior to menstruation, many women crave chocolate. The reason for this is that chocolate contains a significant amount of magnesium, as well as satisfying the immediate energy requirements that blood sugar imbalances induce. But it is better to eat other magnesium-rich foods, such as apricots, figs or peaches, which will satisfy a sweet tooth without leaching away other vital nutrients. Combining any of these foods with a small protein snack such as almonds (which also contain magnesium) or other nuts or seeds will help to balance blood sugar levels.

Polycystic ovarian syndrome ( PCOS ) has become increasingly common. In this condition the ovaries become swollen with fluid-filled sacs, making it difficult for eggs to be released. Nutrition can help to address this syndrome, which is strongly related to excessive production of insulin, which stimulates an enzyme in the ovaries to convert oestrogen into testosterone. This is why women suffering from this syndrome show signs of blood sugar imbalance (irritability, mood swings, headaches, dizziness without food and excessive thirst) and signs of elevated testosterone (weight gain around the abdominal area and increased body hair). Taking dietary steps to address blood sugar imbalances and regain normal insulin secretion often has excellent results.

### nutrition know-how

If you have difficulty sleeping through the night, don't battle with it – get up and prepare yourself a light snack of some dates and bananas, or a low-fat natural yoghurt with a teaspoon of nut butter. Better still, purée a little of all the above in a blender to make a 'midnight milkshake'.

## Is your child wild or mild?

There are several possible causes of hyperactivity in children. Some are linked to genetics or the environment, but by far the most prevalent cause, it appears, is the relationship that the nervous system has with certain foods.

Classic symptoms of hyperactivity include an inability to concentrate on any game or task for more than a few minutes at a time; having excessive spurts of energy followed by exhaustion; head-banging; aggressive behaviour towards other children (and adults); and being easily frustrated and irritated. The child may also be unusually clumsy, restless at mealtimes, and underachieving at school. Repeated attempts at encouraging them to concentrate and focus,

## Foods for memory and concentration

**Whether you're studying hard for exams, spending 10 hours a day in the office, making a presentation, driving a car, or carrying out any activity that requires concentrated brain effort, the food you eat throughout the day will have a direct effect on your ability to concentrate and remember things.**

Brain cells require **choline**, a B vitamin, for optimal function. Once present in the brain, it is transformed into acetyl choline, a neurotransmitter responsible for sending information from one brain cell to the next. Low levels of acetyl choline cause loss of memory in varying degrees – from the 'It's on the tip of my tongue...', to complete forgetfulness. Choline is also required for the formation and maintenance of the myelin sheath that protects the nerve cells, ensuring rapid and accurate transmission of information.

*Choline-rich foods include calf's liver, cabbage, cauliflower, caviar, eggs, lentils and soya products, including tofu.*

Another neurotransmitter, **dopamine**, requires vitamin B3 and iron for its formation. Dopamine is involved in the laying down and maintenance of memory.

*Good food sources of B3 are brewer's yeast, turkey, halibut, pumpkin seeds and peanuts. Iron-rich foods include calf's liver, apricots (particularly when dried), raisins, pumpkin seeds and walnuts.*

**The B-complex vitamins (B1, B2, B3, B5, B6, B12, biotin and B9, folic acid)** are all required for memory maintenance. Signs of deficiency in these vitamins include memory loss, poor concentration, impaired learning and general forgetfulness. B-complex vitamins are essential for the production of cellular energy – and nowhere more than in the brain cells.

*Good food sources include brewer's yeast, chicken, collards, kale, oatmeal, soya beans, fish, avocados and potatoes.*

even for a few minutes at a time, usually prove to be infuriatingly futile.

Food management can help tremendously in controlling hyperactivity. Children respond very quickly to changes in diet and environment, and those foods that are affecting your child will hurriedly make themselves known if you follow a plan of first eliminating the foods from the kitchen for a few weeks, and then re-introducing them. Working with hyperactive children like this is possibly one of the most effective ways of using food as therapy.

The first step is to keep a food diary to determine which foods seem to be having the greatest effect. To monitor changes in behaviour, it is essential to eliminate all sweetened foods, artificial fruit-flavoured drinks, fizzy drinks and squashes and all processed and packaged foods. Foods containing colourings (particularly synthetic blues, greens and oranges), additives and a high level of sugars can all interfere with brain chemistry; this seems to affect some more dramatically than others.

In addition, salicylates (compounds found naturally in some foods, which act like aspirin) have been found to be a major culprit in upsetting the delicate brain chemistry of children. Salicylates are abundant in apricots, almonds, apples, cherries, currants, raisins, all berry fruits, peaches, plums, prunes, tomatoes and oranges. Often, simply removing citrus fruits and orange juice from the diet can have a profound effect on the child's behaviour. Essential fatty acids also play a large part in the management of hyperactivity. Required for

nerve transmission, any imbalance or deficiency in essential fatty acids can affect the sensitive communication from one nerve ending to another. A high-sugar diet can interfere with the utilization of essential fats, causing incorrect or incomplete nerve transmission. Hyperactive children are frequently found to have a deficiency of the omega-3 group of essential fatty acids, and increasing foods that contain them is recommended. Oily fish such as tuna, sardines, salmon and mackerel are all rich in omega-3 fats, as is flax seed oil (which can be used in dressings, but should not be heated).

Green vegetables containing magnesium are often found to be lacking in a hyperactive child's diet, upsetting the fragile calcium–magnesium balance required for optimal brain and nerve function. Serving broccoli, peas, cauliflower, spinach and figs will help to increase intake of magnesium, as will wholegrains, including oats and brown rice.

There can be other causes for hyperactivity in a child. If adjusting your child's diet as discussed above does not make a significant difference to their behaviour, then environmental and toxic elements can be considered. It is advisable to consult a specialist in this field, and there are tests that can be carried out to determine if toxicity is the cause. A nutrition consultant can organise a hair mineral analysis test, which will highlight any heavy metal toxicity that may be contributing to your child's hyperactivity. Other influences include physical trauma, such as a fall, which may have caused unseen damage. Always consult a medical professional for advice.

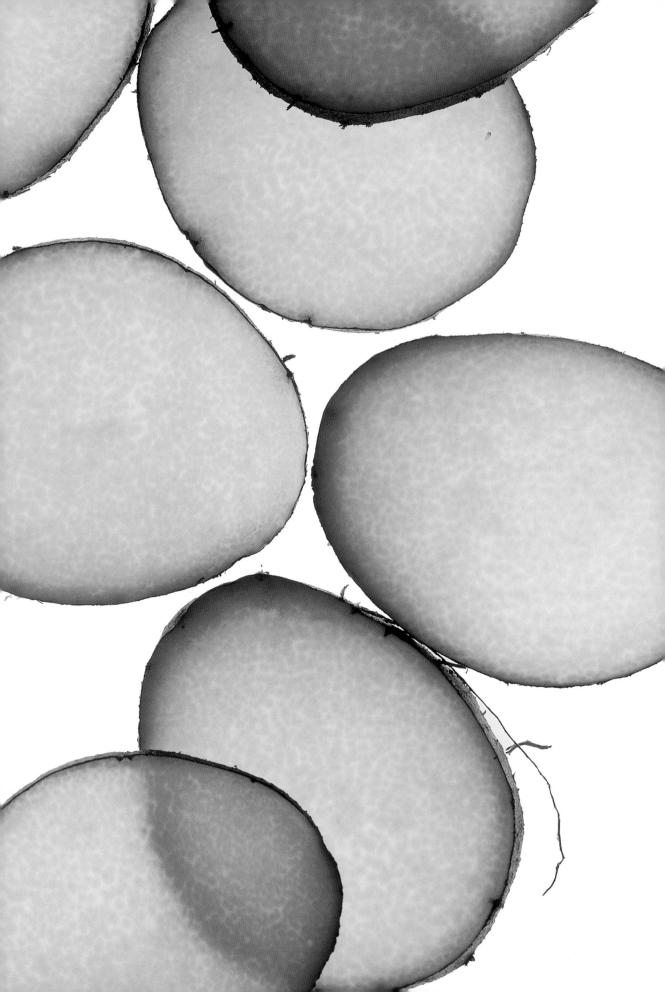

# managing stress

Stress is a modern buzzword, but do you really know what it means? To function as efficiently as possible, the body constantly strives to achieve a perfect balance in all its processes. Stress is any disturbance to that balance. The body has to work hard to combat the physical and emotional stress that it is bombarded with.

Stress is inevitable and can take many forms. It is difficult to imagine a life without it; each of us will find various things stressful at different times. There are two types of stress – external and internal. External (exogenous) stresses, which we are more familiar with, are imposed on the body from outside. Internal (endogenous) stresses occur inside the body. Both are outlined in the box on the right.

## An ancient response to modern stress

To understand how stress can adversely affect the body, we need to look back in time. Early man's ability to survive depended on his skill at hunting and escaping predators. When confronted with the threat of attack, the body instantly reacts by releasing stress hormones that trigger the release of energy to the organs most involved in defending the body. This is called the 'fight or flight' response. Although not frequently confronted by wild animals today, we still react in this way to any perceived threat or challenge. When the hormones are released, the brain becomes more alert and the five senses function with a heightened level of skill.

### Identify your stressors

| External stresses | Internal stresses |
|---|---|
| ● Pollution | ● Food allergies and intolerances |
| ● Hydrogenated fats | ● Auto-immune diseases |
| ● Smoking and alcohol | ● Metabolic waste |
| ● Excessive sun exposure | ● High cholesterol |
| ● Heavy workloads | ● Blood sugar imbalances (and diabetes) |
| ● Emotional problems | |
| ● Bereavement | ● Hormonal imbalances |
| ● Divorce/separation | ● Nutrient deficiencies |
| ● Recreational drugs | ● Depression caused by chemical imbalance |
| ● Medicines | |

At the same time, stored glucose is released from the liver to fuel the skeletal muscles for exertion.

71

LEFT Potatoes are a rich source of vitamin C, which supports the adrenal system.

There are seven major changes that occur in the body when it reacts to stress, all stemming from the 'flight or fight' ability to react to danger. These are:

**1** The heart rate increases to pump extra blood, in order to supply vital nutrients required for energy production.

**2** The breathing rate increases to allow more oxygen into the blood and more carbon dioxide to be excreted.

**3** The spleen produces more blood, carrying with it extra immune cells. The blood itself has a greater ability to clot in case of injury.

As we can see, the 'fight or flight' reaction primes the body for action and is designed to do so for a short, concentrated period of time. But if the body is kept in this heightened state of alarm for long periods, it can damage its physical and emotional well-being. It is like putting your car in neutral and pressing one foot right down on the accelerator and the other on the brakes!

When this occurs, the body seeks to restore its natural balance and harmony, so it adjusts its parameters and adapts to the stress. For example, it may reset blood pressure, allowing it

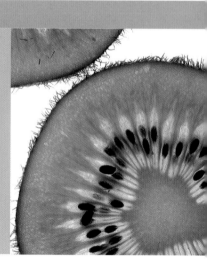

# The long-term effects of stress mean we're constantly living on our nerves – and using up precious energy reserves.

**4** The blood vessels supplying the brain and muscles dilate to allow increased quantities of oxygen, glucose and nutrients to these vital areas.

**5** The liver and skeletal muscles release extra glucose into the blood to provide more energy.

**6** The pupils dilate to allow more light into the eyes to improve vision.

**7** Digestion slows and digestive enzyme secretion is halted, freeing energy for use by the muscles and the brain.

to remain higher than usual, or it may readjust the glucose levels in the blood so that they are continuously being drained. Both, of course, are potentially dangerous.

But, back to the ancestors. After a period of stress, our ancestors rested to allow the body to restore its balance. All the symptoms in the 'fight or flight' response abated, reinstating the normal levels of hormones, blood glucose and digestion. Modern-day life doesn't allow us this luxury of recovery time. Our stresses are so abundant – and frequently continuous – that our bodies end up in a permanent state of 'fight or flight' reaction, without any respite. The long-term result of this is that we remain in high gear, using up our precious stores of glucose and energy. Our bodies never have the chance to rebalance themselves and physiological change can eventually occur. Some of the most common physiological effects of stress are listed below. Added to this, some of the foods we choose to eat also increase the stress on our overtaxed and drained bodies by depleting energy levels and providing insufficient nutrients.

experienced as the body moves into high gear. This is stress in action. However, by the second or third public speaking engagement, initial nerves will have receded and he or she is more likely to approach the task with a sense of calm. Therefore the stress experienced would be much less severe. The situation is the same, it is just the interpretation of it that has altered. If we acknowledge stress and understand that it can be altered, then we can find a way of minimizing it.

## Food as a stressor

Foods that are not particularly good for us or to which we are allergic can cause stress. In

### Stress symptoms – the physiological effects of stress include:

- Food cravings
- Weight loss
- Constant fatigue
- Loss of appetite
- Mood swings
- Immune suppression leading to frequent colds and flu
- Anxiety
- Skin irritation
- Sugar cravings
- Disturbed sleep
- Depression

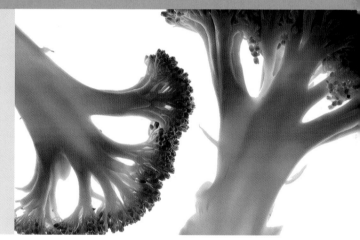

### Interpreting emotional stress

It is an interesting fact that emotional stress is experienced in a uniquely different way by everyone. What may be stressful to you may not be a problem for someone else. The stress of a certain situation may be lessened if we choose to view it differently. Let's use the example of speaking in public, which frightens many people. The very first time someone does this they will probably experience stress: the palms may sweat and an adrenaline rush can be

addition, faulty digestion, induced by poor dietary habits or bacterial or parasitic infections, will increase the likelihood of a leaky gut (see page 87), allowing unwanted food particles to pass into the bloodstream. This causes an immune response, which when it occurs daily overworks the adrenal glands. Ironically, it is a catch-22 situation, as the adrenals respond to stress by releasing increased amounts of another hormone, cortisol, which aims to redress the balance. One of the side-effects of excess or repeated cortisol release is digestive disturbance. The cycle is self-perpetuating – and increasingly damaging to health.

Having a positive outlook on life can also help reduce stress. So what if you are stuck in traffic? It is not your fault so why not listen to some music or talk to your travelling companions. Do what you can to deal with it – use your mobile phone if you have one to tell people why you are late (but not while driving), for example. If you can't do anything, try to accept it.

### Stress, food and nutrition

So what can we do about all this? While we may not be able to influence many of the external factors that induce stress, we can at least help our body to cope with its effects.

Certain nutrients have been shown to help deal with stress and, at the same time, support the organs that are involved in the stress reaction. For example, the Fighting Five – vitamins A, C and E and the minerals zinc and selenium – can disarm the free radicals that are produced if the body is under stress. Foods containing these vital antioxidants include plums, tomatoes, kiwi fruit, dark green vegetables, seafood, sesame seeds and pumpkin seeds.

### Stress and the immune system

It is a well-known and well-documented fact that people affected by stress are more prone to illness. This is due to the dampening effect that long-term stress has on the immune system.

In times of increased stress, we get more colds and infections and, in more serious cases, the body does not deal with pre-cancerous cells with the same efficiency as in times of rest and relaxation. The heightened alertness of the body reduces the immune system's ability to fight infection, as the body deems this to be less important than dealing with the immediate danger it has sensed. The output of the immune system's battling killer cells and T-cells is suppressed, allowing invaders to flourish. As you can see, in periods of stress it is vital to support the immune system.

### Immune system hormones

Two important hormones play a dramatic role in the immune system during periods of stress. These are dehydroepiandosterone (DHEA) and cortisol. Researchers have found that many people suffering chronic conditions have decreased levels of DHEA and increased levels of cortisol (these hormones can easily be measured using a simple saliva test). There are many reasons for the decline in DHEA. Stress acts on the adrenal glands to switch the production of DHEA to that of cortisol. This imbalance can have many consequences for the body, as well as suppressed immunity. DHEA levels decline as we age, and it is thought that we manufacture only 20 per cent as much in our seventies and eighties as we do in our teens and twenties. Declining levels have been linked to increased fat stores (especially around the abdomen), constant hunger, insomnia, lack of interest in sex and an increased incidence of allergies and infections.

If any of these symptoms apply to you, ask your nutritional consultant or health practitioner to test your levels of DHEA and cortisol. If these

When this happens, both hormones may need temporary supplementation, carefully combined with specific herbal nutrients such as licorice, rhodiola and Siberian ginseng. This type of programme would need to be designed and supervised by a professional nutrition consultant.

In the US, it is possible to buy supplements of DHEA from pharmacies and some health food shops. However, in some countries only a doctor can prescribe DHEA or its precursor, pregnenolone, which acts in the same way.

turn out to be low, as soon as adequate levels of DHEA are restored, the benefits will include improved cholesterol levels, increased bone

# Some foods stress the body. A deficiency of any nutrient is a stress in itself, because it places a strain on all the enzyme processes that depend upon it.

health and a better muscle-to-fat ratio. Cortisol can be a dangerous hormone. Increased levels of it are responsible for compromised thyroid function, impaired joint function and decreased energy. Furthermore, a higher amount of cortisol causes the breakdown of muscle and bone, eventually leading to the bone-thinning disease osteoporosis.

### Boosting DHEA and reducing cortisol

The balance of DHEA and cortisol can be restored by supporting the adrenal glands with the foods recommended in Stress-busters (see pages 76–77) and through physical exercise and relaxation techniques such as meditation or yoga.

In the most severe cases of damage caused by long-term stress, the adrenal glands reduce their production of both DHEA and cortisol. This stage is known as adrenal exhaustion or failure.

### Managing stress through diet

So how do we set about managing stress? While it may not be possible to eliminate many of the external stresses that occur in our lives, we do have the power to alter our eating habits and make changes to our lifestyle.

Some foods we eat actually stress the body. A deficiency of any nutrient is a stress in itself, because it places a strain on all the enzyme processes that depend upon it. To support the important adrenal glands, the body needs the following vital vitamins and minerals: vitamin B5, vitamin C and magnesium. To help control the effects of the stress you are subjected to every day, it is essential to include plenty of foods containing these nutrients in your daily diet. The adrenal glands need abundant supplies of vitamin C, a water soluble vitamin that can not be manufactured or stored within the body, so must be obtained daily from our diet. The richest sources include all black and red berries, kiwi fruit, citrus fruits, parsley, watercress, potatoes and peppers – all easily available from supermarkets.

During periods of extreme stress, the requirement for this essential vitamin increases many times over. One of the most common symptoms of vitamin C deficiency is mouth problems such as ulcers (canker sores) and sores. These can be alleviated within 24 hours if optimal levels of the vitamin are supplied.

effect and actually increase stress. Eating high levels of sugars and refined carbohydrates depletes many stored nutrients, especially magnesium, and also puts excessive demands on the pancreas to produce large amounts of insulin (see Blood sugar management, page 60). Over a period of time, the pancreas becomes fatigued and works less efficiently, in some cases leading to the early stages of maturity-onset diabetes.

Cutting or reducing the amount of sugar we eat can have a profoundly beneficial effect on the liver, helping it to perform its detoxification

## Stress-busters

With a demanding work schedule, stopping for a relaxed and nutritious meal is one luxury few people can manage during the day. So in the morning, prepare some nutritious mini-meals to take to work. The following snacks are quick and easy to make and can be eaten 'on the run'.

Smoked mackerel pâté on wholegrain crackers

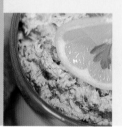

Almond butter on rye toast

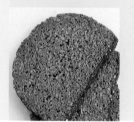

Spinach salad with pumpkin seeds

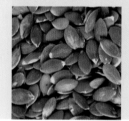

Magnesium is the primary mineral required by the adrenal glands and so magnesium-rich foods should be eaten daily. These include grains, green leafy vegetables, soya beans, sunflower seeds, sesame seeds, wheatgerm, almonds, cod and mackerel. Good sources of vitamin B5 include wholegrains, green leafy vegetables, oranges and animal and dairy products.

So, if certain foods are good for stress, it follows that there are also foods that have a negative

processes more efficiently. The liver is the primary cleansing organ in the body. Its job is to continuously filter the blood to remove all potentially harmful toxins, waste matter and debris produced by natural processes. Reducing any of the stresses put upon the liver will help it to function more efficiently. Stimulant drinks such as tea, coffee and alcohol rob the body of nutrients and encourage the production of adrenaline, so cutting your intake of these is a positive step to controlling your stress.

Needless to say, it is also a good idea to limit, or eliminate, your intake of refined, processed and convenience foods, as they have a lot of artificial preservatives, salt and sugar in them and their nutritional content is usually very, very low.

## Weekend destressing plan

For increased energy, and as a way to detoxify a stressed system, set aside a long weekend when you can allow yourself to do very little. Fill your kitchen with plenty of fresh fruits and vegetables, and limitless mineral water. During the weekend, aim to eat and drink only foods in

particularly beneficial after a bout of excessive eating and/or drinking.

Virtually all vegetables can be juiced, as well as fruits. You should aim to drink between three and four green vegetable juices per day. The best juicing vegetables include watercress, parsley, spinach, courgettes (zucchini), green peppers and lettuce. As fruits are high in fructose, it is advisable to dilute fruit juices 50 per cent with water.

Spend plenty of time resting, go for some gentle walks, and be sure to get lots of sleep. By the

| ...a milkshake with fresh ...ries | Potato salad with rollmop herrings | Strawberry and kiwi fruit salad with soya cream | Mango smoothie with soya milk and sunflower seeds |

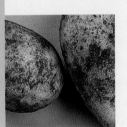
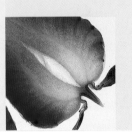
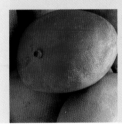

a raw state: these will provide an abundance of nutrients that will help to combat stress.

Start each morning with 3 cups of boiled water, and drink it as hot as you can comfortably stand. You may add either a slice of lemon or 2–3 slices of fresh raw ginger to the water to add flavour, but this should be drunk before anything else. This tonic has a cleansing effect on the liver, and induces the production of bile, to clear any backlog in the common bile duct. This is

second day it is possible that you will experience a headache or some muscle aches and pains, but this is not a bad sign – it shows that your body is detoxifying itself. Remember that you will reap the benefits at the beginning of the following week, when you will feel as if you have been away on vacation! Throughout, ensure that you drink plenty of water. You could also arrange a shiatsu or aromatherapy massage for the second or third days – an enjoyable way to assist the detoxification process.

# managing depression

Depression is not unusual. In fact, it has become so prevalent in the Western world that the names of antidepressant drugs, such as Prozac, are now familiar to most people. Depression and anxiety have many possible causes, but it may surprise you to learn that they can be brought on by a reaction to food.

We all feel depressed from time to time, but we can usually link our unhappiness to an event or set of circumstances. However, many people suffer from depression that has no identifiable cause. This can range from feeling a bit down to being unhappy all the time and, in extreme cases, to not being able to experience any joy in life or to find any reason for living. Feeling down is usually transitory and will improve when life circumstances or mental attitudes change. However, the last three instances are more serious and require attention and treatment.

Food influences our brain chemistry. Some foods promote a feeling of well-being while others can 'bring us down' and suppress positive emotions. Ironically, many of the foods that make us feel good are not especially beneficial to our health, and therefore, as with many areas of nutrition, the aim is to find a healthy balance.

## Carbohydrates and mood

When we eat foods containing carbohydrates and sugar, they encourage the absorption of tryptophan into the brain. Tryptophan is a mood-lifting amino acid that is contained in protein foods. Eating carbohydrates allows tryptophan to be more readily absorbed. Bananas, turkey, cottage cheese and dried dates contain high levels of tryptophan.

All nerve impulses in the brain are carried between the nerve cells by substances known as neurotransmitters. Tryptophan is a precursor to

### Depression checklist

**Use this checklist to discover if you could be suffering from depression**

**Are you:**
- Finding it difficult to get out of bed in the mornings?
- Having problems concentrating?
- Suffering from a recent major loss, or breakdown of a relationship?
- Lacking the energy to participate in things that usually interest you?
- Losing your appetite?
- Craving sweet foods?
- Tearful for no apparent reason?
- Living in a country where sunlight is limited?
- Feeling hopeless, or that there is no point in life?

If you have answered 'yes' to three of more questions, you may be depressed.

Consult your medical doctor and if depression is diagnosed, work with him or her in addition to your nutrition consultant.

the neurotransmitter called serotonin – low levels of which have long been associated with depression and anxiety. Antidepressants such as Prozac affect serotonin levels in the brain. This type of antidepressant belongs to a group of drugs known as Selective Serotonin Re-uptake Inhibitors (SSRIs). These work by inhibiting the re-uptake of serotonin in the brain, allowing it to remain available and so to produce a feeling of well-being.

Vitamin B6 is also involved with the synthesis of serotonin. Ensuring that your diet is rich in foods containing B6 (see chart, right) could help to lift mild depression.

It is no coincidence that when we are feeling depressed, the foods we crave are likely to be sweet ones – ice cream, chocolate or cakes. These foods directly affect brain chemicals. Think what happens when dieting: these carbohydrate-rich foods are removed, inevitably leading to a craving for them – as mood dips and the food cravings become stronger, this ultimately leads to the failure of the diet.

## Dopamine and depression

Dopamine, another brain chemical, acts like a neurotransmitter by helping nerve impulses in the brain cross the tiny gap in between nerve cells. Low levels of dopamine are linked with the incidence of depression, while increased levels can bring about feelings of well-being.

Dopamine is synthesized from tyrosine, an amino acid found in protein foods. It requires the vitamins B12 and B9 (more commonly known as folic acid), as well as the mineral magnesium, for its production.

Foods rich in tyrosine include almonds, avocados, bananas, cottage cheese, lima beans, peanuts (raw and unsalted), pumpkin seeds and sesame seeds. Foods high in vitamin B12 include fish, dairy products and spirulina (although it is not clear whether humans can absorb B12 from spirulina). Those high in folic acid include calf's

## B-vitamin boosters

### Vitamin B1 (thiamine)

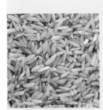

Found in brewer's yeast, brown rice, wheatgerm and soya beans

### Vitamin B3 (niacin or niacinamide)

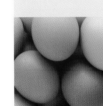

Found in fish, eggs, brewer's yeast, wholegrains and poultry

### Vitamin B6

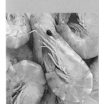

Found in wholegrains such as millet, buckwheat and oats, as well as shellfish such as prawns (shrimp), lobster and mussels

### Vitamin B12 (cyanocobalamine)

Found in fish and dairy products

## The zinc link

The link between zinc levels and depression is a strong one. Very often we see clients with anxiety or depression who show signs of zinc deficiency. Post-partum depression (commonly known as 'the baby blues') has also been attributed to zinc levels, as zinc reserves pass from the mother to the foetus a day or so before birth. Zinc is the basis for the baby's growth and immune system. Replacing the mother's lost zinc after the birth can help conquer depression.

You can carry out a simple test to check if your zinc levels are adequate by answering the questions opposite. If you do decide to increase zinc, no more than 50mg a day should be obtained from all sources (including those provided in a multivitamin supplement). We suggest that you consult a professional nutrition consultant before undertaking any supplementation.

Foods full of zinc include oysters, endives, alfalfa sprouts, seaweed, brown rice, asparagus, mushrooms, turkey and radishes.

## Test your zinc levels

**Check your own zinc levels by answering the following questions.**

**Do you...**

- Have white marks on your fingernails?

- Rarely feel hungry?

- Have pale skin?

- Have stretchmarks around the abdomen or back?

- Have oily skin, perhaps with some acne?

- Suffer from frequent colds or flu?

- Have a poor sense of taste or smell?

If you answer '**yes**' to two or more of these questions, you may well have a deficiency of zinc, in which case we recommend you include some zinc-rich foods in your daily diet. Zinc levels can be more accurately tested by analysing the mineral content of a tiny cutting of hair from the nape of the neck. Most nutrition consultants will be able to arrange this test for you. It is easy to perform and relatively inexpensive.

liver, soya flour, green leafy vegetables (especially broccoli), eggs and brown rice. A good supply of magnesium can be obtained from sunflower seeds, green leafy vegetables, wheatgerm, soya beans, mackerel, swordfish and cod.

### Depression and nutrient deficiency

There is a correlation between levels of some vitamins (especially B-complex) and depression.

Blood plasma levels of these nutrients have been shown to be low in those suffering from depression, and many people have reported that their symptoms improve when they increase their intake of foods with plentiful B vitamins. Vitamin B3 has been shown to be the most effective in managing depression, along with B6 and zinc. Try eating some vitamin B-rich foods every day to see if it helps lift your mood.

## Depression and food allergies

Many clients come to see us for advice on coping with depression. Often, simple food allergies or intolerances are the culprits, and once identified the problem can be remedied easily. Symptoms range from dark circles under the eyes to skin problems, insomnia, irritability, and anxiety.

The trigger foods can be highlighted by a simple blood test. However, in many cases it is easier to remove one or all of the most likely allergens from the diet. In our experience, this process of removal and replacement has shown some remarkable results.

The most common allergens in Europe are wheat, dairy products and citrus fruits, while in the US corn replaces wheat as the most prevalent allergen (see Inflammation, pages 106–113). Many other foods can be responsible, including fast foods or junk foods, colourings and additives. However, we have known of incidences of more unlikely foods being responsible for patients' misery, such as celery or tomatoes.

One example of a food allergy that has a strong link with depression is gluten allergy, which causes coeliac disease (see page 91). If people with this severe sensitivity to all gluten grains do not avoid gluten in their diets, they are more likely to suffer from depression.

While we have seen depressed clients get excellent results by avoiding certain foods, it is still advisable to seek the advice of your doctor if you are depressed, especially if you have been so for a long time.

**nutrition know-how**
Our grandmothers knew that an apple a day was a good thing: this holds true today. Apples contain pectin, which helps to remove lead from the digestive tract – important to those who live in traffic-saturated urban areas.

### Tips for fighting depression

- Poor circulation can decrease the level of oxygen and nutrients required by the brain – so get up and get moving. Circulatory problems are discussed in more depth on page 130.

- You can improve your circulation by eating foods rich in the Fighting Five antioxidants (vitamins A, C, E and the minerals selenium and zinc) found in fresh fruits and vegetables, fish and grains. Iron is also required, as it is essential for the formation of the red blood cells that carry the nutrients in the blood. Offal (organ meats, such as liver), is a rich source of iron, as are apricots and raisins.

- Blood sugar is often a factor in depression (see Blood sugar management, pages 60–64). By learning to choose foods that release their sugars evenly throughout the day, you can avoid the highs and lows of the blood sugar roller-coaster. Eat foods containing complex carbohydrates, found in all grains and vegetables, combined with a small amount of protein from animal foods, dairy produce, nuts or seeds. These will help keep your blood sugar levels balanced all day long.

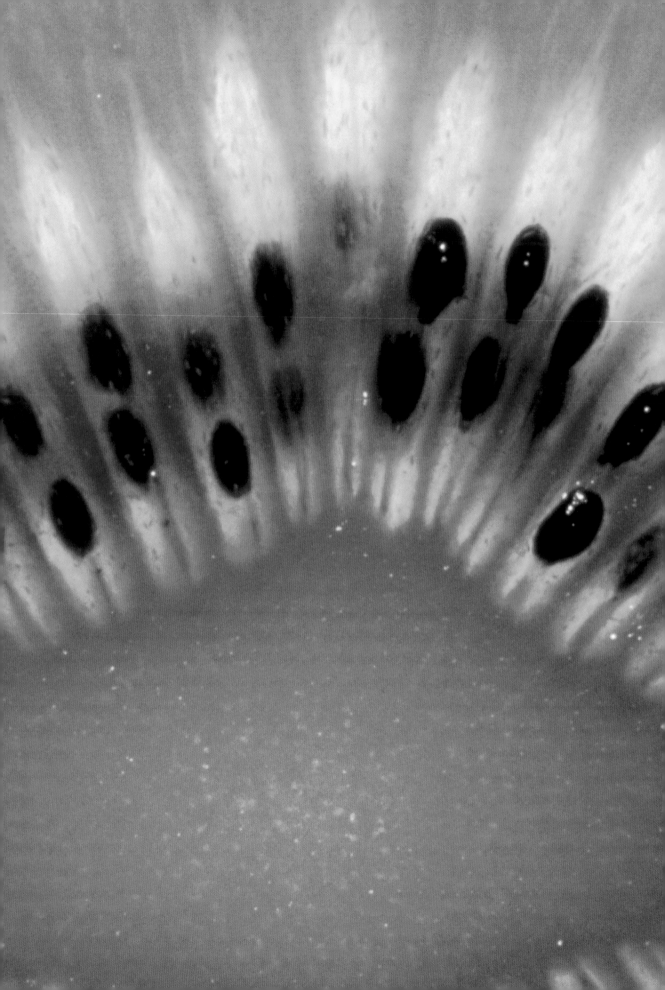

# part two

# Ailments and Remedies

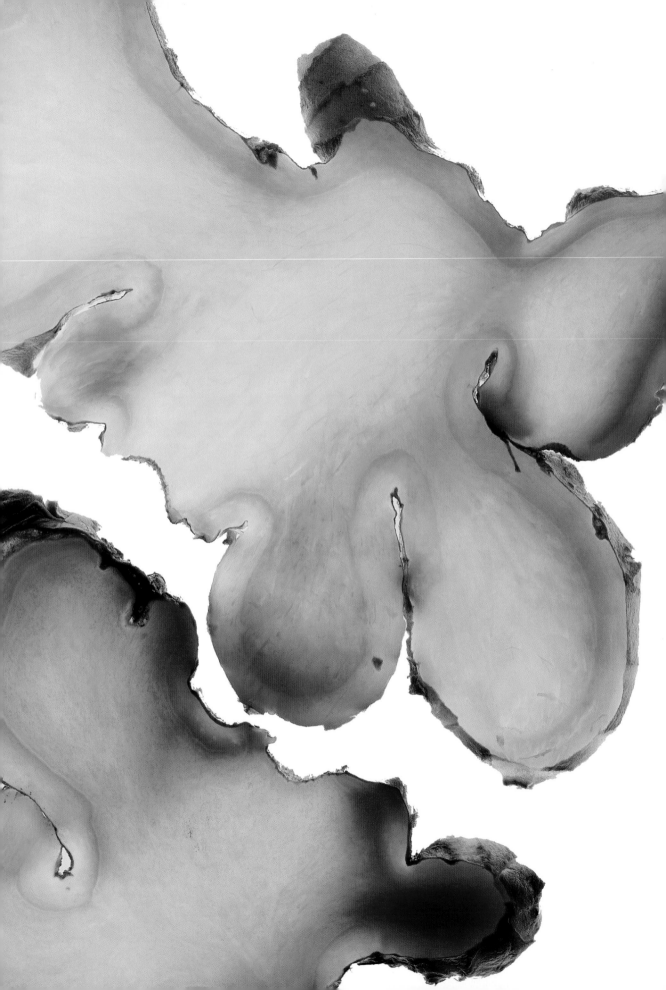

# the digestive system

Digestion is a complicated process that the body carries out virtually continuously – during every minute of the day, whether we're sleeping, working, exercising or resting. Stress, however, interferes with the digestive process, slowing it down or even halting it altogether.

During the 'fight or flight' response, the digestive system shuts down to allow energy to be diverted to where it is more immediately required – for movement, attack or defence. Understanding this shows us how the whole digestive system is put under pressure when we eat 'on the run'.

The type of meals that we eat can also either help or hinder the digestive process. Foods such as fruits, vegetables, wholegrains, nuts, seeds and A-grade proteins (see page 61) promote efficient digestion. A diet high in saturated fats, meat, sugar, caffeine and convenience foods can slow digestion, affecting general health and reducing the absorption levels of essential nutrients.

### The digestive process

In order to understand digestive disorders, we need to know how the digestive system works. The process of digestion starts with the very first thought or smell of food. The brain sends messages to the salivary glands in the mouth to release additional digestive enzymes. This is why you salivate more at the thought of food.

These digestive enzymes are both abundant and powerful, quickly reducing most carbohydrates – such as fruit, vegetables, grains and cereals (granolas) – to a pulp when combined with the chewing process. Meat, nuts and other proteins are more difficult to break down, requiring acid and more specific enzymes, such as those found in the stomach. Thorough chewing is important for crushing solid food particles, increasing the production of salivary enzymes and keeping the teeth clean and sharp. Most people do not chew their food adequately, placing more strain on the digestive system and increasing the likelihood of heartburn and indigestion.

The stomach is pivotal to the whole of the digestive process. It sits behind the ribcage, to the centre of the breastbone. No two people's stomachs are the same: posture, size and height all influence its shape. Sitting upright while eating ensures that the stomach has adequate space to perform its functions. The stomach releases hydrochloric acid, and is the most acidic environment in the body. (Abundant mucus is also produced, to protect the stomach lining

LEFT Ginger helps to quell indigestion and nausea.

from being damaged by its own acid.) The acid gets to work on proteins, while the complex arrangement of stomach muscles contract and relax to churn the food around until it is broken down into partially digested food matter (chyme).

Several factors can adversely affect the production of hydrochloric acid, such as increasing age, recreational and prescription drugs, smoking, alcohol, bacterial infection and stress. This lack of acid can have long-lasting negative effects on digestion and absorption, causing many obvious (and some seemingly unrelated) health problems – see box below.

Hydrochloric acid in the stomach also kills off any ingested bacteria and parasites. It is the first line of defence of the intricate immune system that lines the entire length of the digestive tract. From the age of about 30 onwards, the acid levels tend to diminish, explaining the increasing amount of digestive imbalances and food intolerances that occur as we get older.

An aggressive species of bacteria, *Helicobactor pylori,* can survive in this environment. If untreated, it can cause damage, and therefore requires rigorous antibiotic treatment.

The stomach also produces digestive enzymes. Pepsin further breaks down protein foods, making them easier for the intestines to digest. (Vitamin B6 is required to help this process: consuming plenty of sunflower seeds, kidney beans, barley, broccoli and cauliflower will boost existing levels.) Another enzyme, lipase, starts off the process of digesting fats.

The final process that occurs in the stomach is the binding of vitamin B12 to the intrinsic factor produced in the stomach, allowing it to be absorbed by the intestines. Vitamin B12 is vital for energy production, growth, and the formation of blood and cells.

As we age, levels of intrinsic factor fall, affecting the absorption of vitamin B12 and increasing the possibility of pernicious anaemia (vitamin B12 deficiency). This is why doctors sometimes give B12 injections to people who have been ill, the elderly, or those who are recuperating from surgery. Hydrochloric acid and digestive enzymes will also boost the stomach's own production of vitamin B12, as well as ensuring better protein digestion. To increase your vitamin B12 levels, eat more cottage cheese, haddock, halibut, chicken and tuna.

## Symptoms of faulty digestion

- Burping
- Food allergies
- Indigestion
- Rectal itching
- Iron deficiency
- Nausea

- Bloating
- Headaches
- Vitamin B12 deficiency
- Cracked fingernails
- Intestinal parasites
- Chronic candida

- Stomach upsets
- Constipation
- Gas after meals
- Acne

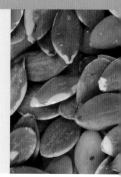

## The small intestine

This is the main area for digestion and absorption. Digestive enzymes that work on fats, proteins and carbohydrates are secreted from the pancreas and further break down the chyme released from the stomach, preparing it for absorption in the three different sections of the small intestine: the duodenum, the jejunum and the ileum. Together, the total length of these sections is about 7 metres (23 feet), but they are all tightly coiled around themselves within the abdominal cavity.

Within the internal face of the three sections, the surface area for digestion and absorption is increased by minute, finger-like projections called villi. These villi secrete enzymes, absorb essential nutrients and prevent food particles and other potentially threatening substances from getting into the bloodstream. This sensitive procedure can be upset by antibiotics and other drugs, alcohol and/or a high intake of sugar. When reacting to such substances, the minute gaps between the cells of the villi become inflamed and widen, allowing unwanted food particles to pass into the bloodstream. This is called intestinal permeability, or a 'leaky gut', and can lead to food intolerances resulting in other immune responses such as headaches, fatigue, skin problems and arthritic types of pain in bone and muscle anywhere in the body.

The duodenum is the entry point for bile, produced in the liver and then concentrated and stored in the gall bladder. Bile is essential for breaking down particles of partially digested fats, allowing them to be absorbed. The pancreas releases bicarbonates to neutralize or reduce the acidity of stomach secretions, and also produces three digestive enzymes – protease to digest protein, lipase for fats and amylase for carbohydrates.

The jejunum and ileum are the major sites for the absorption of the remaining nutrients, including proteins, amino acids, water-soluble vitamins, cholesterol and bile salts.

## The ileo-caecal valve

To separate the small and large intestines and to prevent any faecal matter from passing back up into the small intestine, a tight, one-way valve lies between them. This is the ileo-caecal valve, which is located very close to the appendix. It is an area that can easily become inflamed, as bacteria and parasites often adhere to its walls.

If inflammation occurs over a prolonged period, the ileo-caecal valve may stay open, allowing toxic matter up into the highly absorptive area of the ileum. This can lead to mistaken diagnosis of appendicitis, resulting in the unnecessary removal of the appendix, an important organ of lymphatic tissue. Treatment to kill the parasites or bacteria, and the removal of any potentially irritating foods (such as grains, pulses [legumes] and large amounts of fibre) for a short period, can remedy this minor problem without the need for invasive procedures.

## The large intestine

The large intestine, also known as the colon, is made up of three consecutive sections (the ascending, transverse and descending colon), ending in the rectum and anus. Its muscular structure contracts and relaxes every few seconds to move the remaining matter – water, bacteria, insoluble fibre and waste products derived from the digestion process – towards the anus. This waste material is known as faeces.

Right from the start, when a mouthful of food is swallowed, the whole digestive process relies on a series of muscle contractions and relaxations called peristalsis to move food through the system, rather like the way a snake moves across the ground. The muscles that carry out peristalsis are heavily dependent on two minerals – calcium and magnesium – for efficient functioning. An imbalance between these two minerals can result in bowel problems such as constipation or diarrhoea.

It is important to recognize the urge to go to the toilet and respond to it, as holding back faecal matter for even a couple of hours causes a greater absorption of water, which results in drier and more constipated stools. This is one of the main causes of haemorrhoids.

It is 'normal' to have at least one bowel movement a day. Those with an efficient digestive system may 'go' after every meal. It is not uncommon, however, for several days to pass without a bowel movement, allowing toxic waste matter to be reabsorbed through the intestinal wall back into the bloodstream. This is a frequent cause of fatigue, headaches, nausea and feeling under the weather, explaining why a doctor will always ask a patient about bowel movements, even for a seemingly unrelated ailment. The problems related to constipation are discussed further on.

### A healthy large intestine

To keep the large intestine healthy and functioning, you should eat vegetables, fruit and insoluble fibre (derived from grains and pulses [legumes]) every day. These foods all contain magnesium, which keeps the muscles of the large intestine functioning well. While drinking juices made from liquidized fruit and vegetables provides an excellent source of magnesium, you should still eat several helpings per day of each in their whole form, as it is their fibrous content that helps to remove toxic waste matter from the large intestine, as well as encouraging regular muscle contraction and relaxation.

People who undergo any form of abdominal surgery have to be very careful with what they eat after the operation, as the natural process of elimination can be seriously disturbed for several days. Patients should be given simple meals for the first couple of days which do not tax the large intestine, decreasing the likelihood of constipation. Vegetable soups, salads, lightly steamed vegetables and rice are the best foods at this time as they are nutritionally rich, easily digested and absorbed and contain the necessary fibre to stimulate the colon's return to normal functioning.

### Digestive immunity

Between 60 and 70 per cent of the body's immune system is in the digestive tract – but this is not surprising if you consider the multitude of potentially harmful substances and bacteria that enter the body through the first part of the digestive system: the mouth. There are billions of protective bacteria living in the mouth, oesophagus and small intestine, and literally trillions in the large intestine. As the stomach is such a highly acidic environment, fewer protective bacteria are required, since most invaders cannot survive there.

Some 400–500 different types of bacteria have been identified in the gut, some of which are anti- and some pro-cancerous; some that synthesize vitamins B, A and K; some that produce substances to fight specific infections; and others that digest lactose (milk sugars) and regulate muscle contraction and relaxation. They produce natural antibiotics and anti-fungals to prevent the growth of unwelcome bacteria and fungus, as well as breaking down the toxic waste produced by invading bacteria, which is potentially more harmful than the bacteria themselves. They do this by producing large amounts of acid.

The protective bacteria also play an important role in guarding against the potentially harmful effects of toxic metals that get into the body, such as mercury from amalgam fillings and contaminated fish, radiation (from anti-cancer treatment; also found in some foods), and the pesticide and herbicide residues in most non-organic produce. Some bacteria are also

responsible for manufacturing hydrogen peroxide, in the presence of which cancer cells cannot survive. However, there are many factors that can disrupt the balance of these essential bacteria, as outlined in the box below.

The protective gut bacteria will remain dominant in the digestive tract, provided that it is a friendly environment undisturbed by an accumulation of harmful factors (see below). If, however, you are eating a poor diet, consuming alcohol regularly, living under constant stress, using antacids and painkillers on a frequent basis, or taking frequent courses of antibiotics prescribed by your doctor, that delicate balance will be thrown out. The 'bad' bacteria then have a chance to override the beneficial bacteria.

This type of lifestyle is very common – in fact, for many people, it is normal. Those who identify with it will also suffer from frequent indigestion, bloating and gas – and wonder why. The answer is simple. Their intestinal bacteria are at war.

Over the next six pages, we will examine a number of common digestive diseases in a little more detail.

## Lifestyle factors affecting digestive efficiency

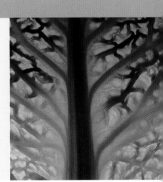

| | | |
|---|---|---|
| ● Antibiotics | ● Anti-inflammatories | ● Stress |
| ● High-fat diet | ● Fried foods | ● Bereavement |
| ● Sugar | ● Alcohol | ● Smoking |
| ● Processed foods | ● Canned drinks (sodas) | ● Recreational drugs |

# digestive conditions

### Bloating and wind

It is not uncommon to suffer from a painful, bloated or distended stomach after eating, and there are a few reasons why this could be happening. Lack of stomach acid and/or digestive enzymes means that the food you eat does not get fully digested, setting the scene for food intolerances and mild intestinal inflammation, and resulting in bloating. Stress, eating on the run and not chewing your food properly all reduce stomach acid and digestive enzyme output. If this is relevant to you take a few minutes to relax before eating, eat slowly remembering to chew well, and eat away from your desk at work.

The large intestine plays host to a multitude of bacteria, yeasts and occasional parasites. These microbes are capable of feasting on undigested foods, proteins and sugar, producing gas or wind as a by-product of their fermentation. If your diet is high in sugar and protein whilst being low in fibre (lacking fresh vegetables and pulses (legumes), then this fermentation may be responsible for your bloating and wind. Cutting out sugar and reducing animal protein in your diet along with supplementing your diet with a 'probiotic' (capsules of beneficial gut bacteria) may help to restore bowel function.

For some people the smooth muscles of the intestine go into a mild spasm after eating. This whips the contents of the intestine into a foam, creating trapped wind. Essential oil of peppermint can relax these muscles, dispersing the foam and releasing the trapped wind, so sip fresh peppermint tea after meals to soothe a grumbling stomach.

### Constipation

The main cause of constipation is dehydration. Also, constipation is one of the foremost reasons for frequent headaches. It is essential to drink 1.5–2 litres (3–4 pints) of still mineral water every day to satisfy the body's minimum requirements and to prevent constipation. If exercising, this intake should be doubled. Other causes of constipation are a high-protein diet without sufficient vegetable fibre, and a high intake of alcohol, tea, coffee and caffeinated drinks, all of which are dehydrating.

To avoid constipation, it is essential that the diet contains lots of soluble fibre, derived from fruits and vegetables, plus insoluble fibre from rice, barley, buckwheat and other grains. (If you are constipated and not drinking enough liquids, pulses (legumes) will only exacerbate the problem, causing solids to build up.)

Constipation is more common during pregnancy and is often caused by taking iron supplements. Eating dried apricots that have been soaked overnight tackles both of these problems, as apricots are one of the highest fruit sources of iron and are also mildly laxative. However, if you are pregnant, do not stop taking iron tablets in order to replace them with natural sources unless you have the agreement of your doctor.

### Candida

This is a much talked-about problem affecting a large number of people. It is not well understood, but is thought to be mainly due to diet and lowered immunity. *Candida albicans* is naturally present in the digestive tract and is not harmful unless the immune system is compromised or a high-sugar diet is consumed. If this happens, it mutates into a potentially damaging fungus. The first signs of candida overgrowth include bloating, excessive gas and abdominal cramps that occur after eating fruit and other sweet foods. If the condition continues unchecked, it can lead to serious fatigue and mild depression. Some of the less obvious symptoms of candida overgrowth include insomnia, itchy ears, aching shoulders, irritability, lack of concentration, sore throat, muscle pain, hyperactivity and acne.

One of the main causes of candida overgrowth is the frequent use of antibiotics. While they are essential for stamping out persistent infections, antibiotics also kill off all the bacteria in the gut, including protective bacteria. This allows *Candida albicans* to multiply – often described as a 'yeast overgrowth'. See the Lifestyle Questionnaire on page 8 for information on the relationship between yeast overgrowth and various health problems.

## Coeliac disease

Coeliac disease is a disease of the intestines in which the villi (the tiny hair-like protrusions that absorb nutrients from food) are flattened after coming into contact with gluten. Coeliac disease can cause malnutrition, diarrhoea, weight loss or just a general failure to thrive. This condition is quite common and is thought to run in families. In babies, it will usually manifest itself within a few weeks of the infant being introduced to solids containing gluten, but it can be triggered off at any stage in life.

Sufferers are allergic to gluten in all forms, so they should avoid wheat, barley, oats and rye. The traditional treatment for coeliac disease required the cutting out of all starches and grains, including rice, potatoes and corn, in addition to gluten. Some people still do this, although nowadays it is not thought to be necessary. Many sufferers maintain an excellent level of health, as their diets tend to include a large proportion of fresh fruit and vegetables, as well as fish, chicken and gluten-free grains.

## Diarrhoea

There are many possible causes of diarrhoea and it is more likely to be a symptom of another problem than a condition in itself. However, acute diarrhoea is usually the result of an infection. Bloody diarrhoea is a sign of serious inflammation and you should see your doctor.

Intermittent bouts of diarrhoea may be caused by food allergies, parasitic infections, excessive caffeine consumption, pancreatic problems or stress levels. If your diarrhoea started after a trip abroad and is frequently accompanied by stomach pains then you may have picked up a parasite. A nutrition consultant or your doctor can arrange for a stool test to check for any intestinal infections.

Diarrhoea robs the body of large amounts of water, and with it valuable minerals. Always make sure you replace these after an attack by eating mineral-rich foods such as nuts, green vegetables and perhaps seaweed. Lost potassium must be replaced at once: abundant sources are avocados, chard, lentils, parsnips, spinach, most fresh nuts, sardines and bananas.

If you occasionally get diarrhoea, the culprit may well be food, so change your diet and monitor whether or not there is an improvement. If there is not, consider consulting a nutrition consultant and/or your doctor.

### Food poisoning

Food poisoning occurs when a toxic substance is consumed, most often some form of bacteria. Symptoms can be apparent within a few minutes of ingesting the offending food, although it can take up to one week for some strains of bacteria to manifest themselves. This makes it less likely that the sufferer will attribute the illness to the guilty food. So it is quite possible that food contamination is more widespread than is currently believed.

There are numerous strains of food-poisoning bacteria, ranging from *Salmonella typhimurium* and *Escherichia coli* (*E. coli*) to *Clostridium botulinum*. Symptoms of food poisoning include chills, fever, chronic diarrhoea and muscle paralysis. There may well be frequent nausea and vomiting as well.

If you suspect that you may have been affected by contaminated food, seek medical advice. Nutritional aids to recovery include garlic, a powerful detoxifier, and potassium-rich foods, such as fruits and green leafy vegetables, to help replace lost minerals. Live bio yoghurt should help to re-establish the beneficial bacteria that live in the gut. Charcoal tablets (from health food shops) can minimize the effects of many toxins, so take them at the first sign of poisoning. Reduce the likelihood of food poisoning by taking sensible precautions. If you have any concerns about a food, then do not eat it! However, taking a garlic tablet before eating can help to detoxify pathogens. While you have little control over what a restaurant serves you, at home you can take avoidance measures. Follow the food hygiene tips listed in the box below.

### Basic food hygiene

- Wash your hands before handling food and after handling raw meat.

- Always keep food hot or cold, not at room temperature.

- Ensure that all cooked foods are evenly and thoroughly heated.

- If eating outdoors, ensure that the food is well chilled and then eaten immediately after it is set out. Do not allow the food to sit in the sun.

- Do not buy food in cans that are damaged or swollen, even if the store is offering them at a bargain price. No amount of discount is worth the risk of severe food poisoning.

- Do not let raw meat come into contact with other foods during storage or preparation. Keep two or three separate chopping boards specifically designated for different foods.

## Heartburn and indigestion

Heartburn is characterized by pain that appears to rise from the stomach towards the throat, together with a feeling of acidity. Indigestion is similar, but the sensation is static. The traditional treatment for heartburn and indigestion is to take an antacid, yet this does carry some risk, as continued use of antacids disturbs the delicate acid–alkaline balance (pH) of the body and increases the risk of aluminium toxicity. The buffering systems that the body employs to rebalance pH become stressed, and if combined with a high-protein diet the kidneys can be damaged.

We see many clients whose condition is attributable to diet. If you are prone to indigestion or heartburn, try simplifying your meals. If you are eating many proteins, raw and cooked foods at one sitting, it can overload the digestive system. Foods should be eaten slowly and properly chewed. Avoid swallowing anything scalding hot or freezing cold. Caffeine, spicy foods, alcohol and sugar are all known to be stong stomach irritants. If you have continued problems, visit your nutrition consultant, because a food intolerance or enzyme deficiency could be involved. If you suddenly develop indigestion which is severe and persistent, you should check with your doctor to rule out serious causes.

## Hiatus hernia

A hiatus hernia occurs when the stomach bulges up into the chest, allowing food from the stomach to go back up into the oesophagus. Symptoms include heartburn, indigestion, belching and a burning sensation due to stomach acid coming into contact with the delicate oesophagal membrane which, in the long term, can cause oesophageal ulcers.

Drinking aloe vera juice twice a day will help soothe the area. This can be bought in most health food shops and the flavoured variety is usually the most palatable. Zinc is essential for tissue repair; good food sources are pumpkin seeds, wholegrains, eggs, turkey and shellfish such as oysters, lobsters, mussels and crabs.

## Haemorrhoids

With haemorrhoids, the veins around the anus become enlarged. This common condition can be the cause of much pain and discomfort. Symptoms include anal swelling, irritation, burning and some bleeding. (Always remember, blood in stools should be seen by a doctor.)

A diet low in fibre and water can be responsible for haemorrhoids, as straining to defecate causes unnecessary pressure on the veins. Boosting fibre by eating more green vegetables and whole grains will soften faeces and make them easier to pass. Calcium and magnesium-rich foods assist healing. Good sources include vegetables, nuts and seeds. Severe, debilitating haemorrhoids require medical treatment.

## Irritable bowel syndrome

It is estimated that as many as 15 per cent of the population of the UK and 20 per cent of the US population suffer from irritable bowel syndrome (IBS). With IBS, the movement of the digestive tract is disturbed, upsetting its natural rhythm. The passage of food is therefore interrupted, and this leads to a build-up of toxins and waste.

Symptoms of IBS include pain, bloating and intermittent bouts of diarrhoea and constipation. Malabsorption of nutrients is also common.

It is important to restore natural muscle tone in the gut, and the B-complex vitamins are most useful for this. These can be found in wholegrains, fish, eggs and wheatgerm. Eating live bio yoghurt daily can help to promote the growth of friendly gut bacteria – this is vital for the digestive system, and also the synthesis of B vitamins. It is believed that sufferers of IBS require higher amounts of protein: A-grade protein sources such as tofu, fish and chicken are best.

**nutrition know-how**

Apples stimulate the growth of beneficial bacteria in the large intestine. They also contain pectin, which helps remove excess cholesterol and toxic metals from the digestive tract.

these have side-effects – see page 93), or drinking large quantities of water to dilute the acid and so reduce the pain. Cabbage is also a fantastic tonic for the stomach and small intestine lining. This vegetable helps re-establish good levels of protective mucus, protecting and healing the delicate cells. A great way to include this into your diet is to drink fresh cabbage and apple juice on a daily basis until symptoms improve. Cabbage juice is also rich in the amino acid methionine which supports liver detoxification and accelerates healing.

Avoiding processed foods, salt, spices, coffee and fried foods should offer some relief from pain and work to prevent future attacks. It is better to have frequent small meals throughout the day, consisting of wholegrains, steamed vegetables and a little A-grade protein, rather than three large meals. As with heartburn, someone developing severe acid pain, especially if over 30 and losing weight, should consult their doctor in order not to miss a serious cause.

### Peptic/duodenal ulcer

In this painful condition, the lining of the stomach or duodenum is eroded, leading to irritation of the tissues. The key symptom is a burning pain, especially one that comes on after eating. Ulcers are associated with stress, because stress can adversely affect stomach acid levels. Another factor to be ruled out with ulcers is the presence of the bacterial infection *Helicobacter pylori*, which can survive in the stomach and contributes to inflammation and erosion of the stomach lining. A nutrition consultant or your doctor can test for this bacteria and treat as necessary. Remedies include taking antacids (but

### Crohn's disease

Crohn's disease can affect both the small and large intestines, causing inflammation, thickening and ulceration. The symptoms include weight loss, frequent and severe diarrhoea, persistent stomach distention and apparent food intolerances manifesting as chronic fatigue, aching muscles, skin rashes and acne. In severe cases, surgical removal of parts of the small intestine may be required.

Nutritional management can be highly effective. This usually requires the omission of wheat and dairy products to reduce inflammation and excess mucus. Other food intolerances are usually found to aggravate the disease, including citrus fruit, tomatoes, spicy food, black peppercorns, coffee, cola drinks and alcohol, so these have to be screened out.

The most important area to address is the inflammation caused by Crohn's disease. During the first few months it is essential to reduce the intake of insoluble fibre, so less fruit should be eaten, particularly those containing small pips, such as strawberries and kiwi fruit, which can be irritating to the digestive tract. A bland diet that includes skinned potatoes, steamed fish, poultry, soft vegetables such as courgettes (zucchini), spinach, peas, butternut squash and wild yam can be particularly beneficial.

Fish should constitute the main source of protein, because they contain anti-inflammatory omega-3 essential fatty acids and vitamin E, which is both an antioxidant and a tissue-healing promoter. Foods rich in zinc are also vital for their healing properties. These foods include poultry, eggs and seafood (which also contains selenium, an antioxidant). Wholegrains, although they are a good source of zinc, should be omitted until all symptoms have abated.

### Ulcerative colitis
The colon is the site of this painful condition, which causes ulcers to erupt. Typical symptoms include severe bloody diarrhoea, mucus in the faeces and acute pain.

Although fibre is needed, only one particular type is appropriate. We, as well as other nutritionists, recommend reducing insoluble

fibre (found in foods such as sweetcorn, and high-starch vegetables such as carrots, turnip, parsnips and swede [rutabaga]), because it is difficult to digest if you have this condition. Avoid wholegrains. Boiled white rice, which has a soothing effect on the digestive tract, can be eaten, especially if cooked with a little garlic. Nuts and seeds are too irritating, so avoid these. All simple carbohydrates and sugars should also be eliminated from the diet – these include bread, biscuits, cakes, pies and pasta. Wheat may be aggravating and may hinder the healing of the intestinal tract, so check foods for wheat content.

Sufferers find that eating small meals frequently throughout the day, rather than three main meals, is easier on the digestive tract. For the same reason, the evening meal should be kept light. Good foods to eat include those rich in soluble fibre such as fruit, green leafy vegetables and their juices, especially parsley, watercress, cabbage, collards and spinach. These will provide the body with fibre without being too abrasive.

Vitamin E is essential for the healing process, so eat plenty of avocados, kale and yams, which will help calm inflammation and soothe ulceration. Omega-3 essential fatty acids are anti-inflammatory, and can be found in oily fish such as salmon, tuna, herrings, sardines and mackerel. Sunflower and pumpkin seed oils will also help. Buy cold-pressed oils and do not heat them.

Both Crohn's disease and ulcerative colitis are very serious diseases which can have life-threatening complications. Any nutritional manipulation should be carried out in combination with conventional medical care.

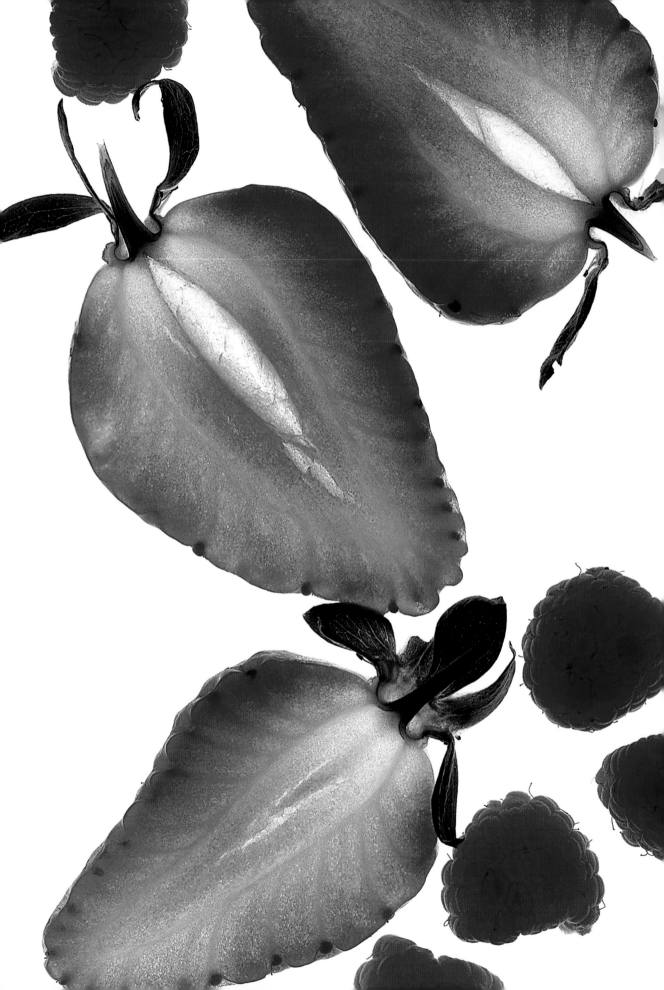

# the immune system

The immune system is perhaps the most intricate of the body systems. It spends almost all its time dealing with potentially harmful invading particles. As you read this, the chances are that your immune system is doing battle with an army of pathogens (harmful tiny organisms, such as bacteria or viruses).

Pathogens are everywhere – in the air, on surfaces, in food and in water. They can be found on our bodies, lurking on skin, hair and under our nails. They also get inside us. If the immune system is not functioning at peak levels, these pathogens can precipitate an infection.

But how often do we think about looking after our immune system? Most people know that it is a good idea to take a vitamin C supplement and drink more orange juice when they have a cold, but that is about the extent of their knowledge. Although understanding exactly how the immune system operates is a lifetime's work, it is important to grasp the basics, so that you know how nutrition and lifestyle can help or hinder your immunity. Meanwhile, find out how good your immune system is by answering the questions in the quiz on page 98.

### Basic defence

The body has some cunning defence systems to guard it against harm. The very first line of defence is the skin, which forms a barrier around us. Its surface is protected by sebum, an oily layer that inhibits the growth of some bacteria. Sweat glands within the skin also assist in fighting off tiny, potentially harmful microbes, by releasing perspiration to help wash them away from the skin's surface.

The tear ducts in our eyes help eliminate possible pathogenic bacterial invaders by producing extra fluid in an effort to flush away offending particles. Hayfever sufferers are acutely aware of this reaction during the summer months, when pollen counts are high and the eyes struggle to repel irritant grains of pollen with streaming tears.

The air that we breathe contains many malevolent particles, which the respiratory tract works to combat. The internal skin (epithelium) of the respiratory tract is lined with tiny, hair-like protrusions (cilia), which trap and collect foreign particles. The secretion of mucus increases in order to help trap pathogens – a substance called secretory immunoglobin A (sIgA), found in mucus, has the ability to neutralize invaders.

LEFT Berry fruits are high in vitamin C and help to strengthen immunity.

## Immune system quiz

**How efficient is your immune system? Testing yourself with the following questions will give you an indication.**

1  Do you often get colds, sniffles or flu?

2  If you have a cold, is it hard to get rid of?

3  Do you frequently feel stressed?

4  Do you suffer from depression or anxiety?

5  Are you allergic to any foods?

6  Do you use painkillers on a regular basis?

7  Do you suffer from hayfever?

8  Have you used antibiotics more than once in the last year?

9  Do you suffer from sore throats?

10 Do you drink alcohol more than three times a week?

11 Do you often get headaches?

- If you have answered **'yes' to three questions**, your immune system may well need some support.
- If you have answered **'yes' to four questions**, it is much more likely that your immune system requires attention.
- Answering **'yes' to five or more** shows that your system is probably over-taxed.

The saliva in the mouth helps flush away microbes that are either airborne in origin or have entered attached to food. When the saliva is swallowed, it mingles with gastric fluid in the stomach which contains a strong acid called hydrochloric acid (see pages 85–86). This destroys most of the bacteria that has been ingested. Some bacteria, however, such as *Helicobacter pylori*, are not destroyed. If microbes do manage to get as far as our intestines, the beneficial flora (bacteria) living there should combat the invaders.

In short, the whole body has some protection on the outside and the inside. Sometimes, however, despite the body's best efforts, harmful invaders do break through the body's defence system and cause illness.

## The immune force

So what does happen when we ingest or inhale a potentially harmful microbe or pathogen? The 'immune force' which protects us is rather like a naval fleet surrounding an island – the body. The fleet protects us from the outside world and is also responsible for detecting and clearing away debris and cells that are behaving unusually, such as cancerous cells. Commanders in strategic positions control individual craft and direct them into battle where required.

The fleet is made up of immune cells. Some of them sail through the body on the lookout for foes, while others have set positions and attack enemies that happen to pass by them. The wandering cells are known as macrophages, and have the ability to destroy and digest pathogens, a process that is known as phagocytosis (see page 100). Immune cells are generally carried in the blood. There are two types of blood cell, red and white, and each has different tasks.

## Red blood cells

These are the most plentiful immune cells in the body. They are synthesized in bone marrow, from where they are released into the bloodstream. The primary role of red blood cells is to carry and deliver oxygen around the body, but they also have the ability to attract pathogens which, in turn, draws the attention of the white blood cells. Red blood cells have a short lifespan, and once they are no longer effective they are filtered out and broken down.

## White blood cells

There are several types of white blood cell and their role is to defend the body. Certain white cells deal with parasitic and allergic reactions such as hayfever and asthma, while others cope with inflammation and infections.

The T-helper cell is an important white blood cell. When it senses the presence of a pathogen, it acts as an early-warning system, alerting the body's immune system defenders to launch an attack on the invader. In cases of HIV, it is these T-helper cells that are diminished, causing the immune system to fail to react to an invasion.

## Complement and interferon

Complement (see page 111) and interferon are also part of the immune navy. They resemble additional marine forces, which the navy can send for when it needs some back-up. They have specific targets and are called upon when other parts of the immune system recognize particular pathogens. Complement is specifically involved with the destruction of tumour cells and disarming some viruses, such as *Herpes simplex*. Interferon is a substance that is secreted by most tissue as a means of self-defence, once it has been affected by a pathogen. It has antiviral properties and relies directly upon vitamin C and the mineral manganese: this is why additional vitamin C is so necessary during the treatment of colds and flu.

## Tracking an infection

In order to see how the immune system functions, let's track the progress of an infection to see how it sets about causing illness.

Imagine you are sitting with friends in a café, enjoying breakfast. The person on the next table sneezes. Minute droplets are sprayed into the air at speeds up to 100 mph (185 kph). They are, for only a few seconds, infectious. As luck would have it, you inhale. The infectious agent that caused your breakfast neighbour to sneeze has now found a new host – you.

Your immune system swings straight into action: first, your nose tries to trap and neutralize the pathogen. If this fails, the pathogen enters the body tissue, where it damages cells, releasing substances usually held within them, such as histamine. This is part of the process of inflammation, described in detail on pages 106–113. The release of histamine alerts white blood cells (see page 99), which travel to the affected tissue and begin their work of destroying the pathogen. Now the pathogen is damaged, and its own cells leak antigens, which attract the attention of the B-lymphocytes. These set about manufacturing 'nets' to trap and engulf the pathogen, effectively disarming it by making it visible to the macrophages, which come along and digest the invader. During this process, you would probably experience a rise in temperature as your body resets its internal thermometer to disable the pathogen. You might have a sore throat, a blocked nose and headaches – all the classic symptoms of a cold.

But what of your companions at breakfast? Perhaps they were infected too, perhaps not. The strength (or weakness) of the immune system underlines our biochemical individuality. Someone whose immune system has been lowered by poor nutrition and immunosuppressors such as sugar and alcohol may develop the cold, whereas someone with a strong immune system is likely to be relatively unaffected, because the mobilized immune fleet will deal with the infection promptly.

## nutrition know-how

For the perfect immune-boosting lunch, why not try the delicious warm turkey and watercress salad on page 154? This will provide ample vitamin C, together with magnesium, calcium, potassium and beta-carotene.

For each person, the pathogen remains the same, but the territory it encounters differs. We will now look at how best to provide your immune system with the nutrition that it requires.

### Nutrition and the immune system

While the immune force is battling a cold virus, it is likely that other pathogens are trying to invade the body at the same time. The constant threat of infection puts the immune force under tremendous pressure, and we must help it by ensuring that it is supplied with all the nutrients necessary for peak fighting performance. Feeding the troops must be the highest priority.

### Vitamin C

Vitamin C is perhaps the most important vitamin for the health of the immune system. It has potent antiviral properties, which is important because viruses, even when dormant, have been shown to undermine immunity. Its role as a support for interferon and complement has already been discussed (see page 99).

Vitamin C is also antibacterial: it detoxifies bacteria and prevents them from replicating. In addition, it is essential for the process of disarming and devouring invading pathogens, carried out by the immune cells, which stimulate the production of specific antibodies. This process is enhanced by the presence of zinc.

Vitamin C and sulphur are needed for the production of strong collagen and connective tissue, which separate and line different areas of the body. Weak collagen and connective tissue allow pathogens easy access to spread between organs and body tissue. Good vitamin C levels help to form the strength of connective tissue needed to keep infections contained in localized areas within the body.

The important, positive effects that vitamin C has on immunity must not be underestimated. When the immune system is undermined, it is critically important to meet the increased need for this vital nutrient. When in good health, an adult needs 1000–2000 mg per day of vitamin C. This requirement can double or treble when the immune system is compromised.

The body cannot manufacture its own vitamin C, so it must obtain an adequate supply each day through diet and nutritional supplements. Rich natural sources include strawberries, kiwi fruit, watermelon, watercress, parsley and sweet potatoes. If your diet contains plenty of fruit and vegetables, you should be getting enough vitamin C. However, if you drink a lot of alcohol, smoke, are under stress, or are at a time when your immune system needs particular support, the vitamin C provided by food may require additional supplementation. One way to gauge whether the body has reached its vitamin C limit is the bowel tolerance test. Diarrhoea indicates that cells have been flooded with vitamin C, so the dose should be cut by half.

### Vitamin A

The immune system needs adequate supplies of vitamin A in order to function well, because it has potent antiviral properties. Vitamin A is important for the health of mucus membranes, such as those found in the nose, throat, mouth, lungs and vagina, as these surface areas are constantly in battle with invading pathogens. Plentiful amounts of vitamin A exist in red and yellow fruits and vegetables, such as carrots, peaches and pumpkins; also in green vegetables such as broccoli. Plus it is found in hard cheese, eggs and liver. Pregnant women should not take vitamin A supplements, or eat liver, unless advised to do so by their doctor.

### Vitamin B6

The white cells' ability to eat up offending pathogens is enhanced by this vitamin. Furthermore, the thymus gland requires good levels of B6. Food sources include brown rice, brewer's yeast and green vegetables.

### Magnesium

This vital mineral is often lacking from the diet. In the context of immunity, magnesium is involved in the synthesis of complement (see page 99), and is essential in ensuring proper thymus function. Magnesium is also required for the formation of prostaglandins (hormone-like compounds found in all tissues) and for controlling histamine levels (see page 110). Magnesium is found in dark green vegetables, fish, soya beans and sesame and pumpkin seeds.

### Calcium

Another vital mineral, calcium plays many roles in the immune system. Firstly, it is involved in the synthesis of the enzymes that T-cells use to defeat pathogenic invaders. Like vitamin C, it is essential for enabling the white cells to digest and destroy certain viruses. Complement is also dependent on adequate calcium in the body. Although high levels of calcium are found in dairy products, these usually contain a lot of saturated fats which are considered to be pro-inflammatory and therefore detrimental to the immune system. It is better to get calcium from

### Iron

Iron can be both helpful and detrimental to the immune system. It plays an essential role in the production of all white blood cells, and is involved in the synthesis of antibodies. However, if too much iron is present, bacteria will thrive. This is not to say that during an infection iron-rich foods should be excluded from the diet. However, supplements containing iron should not be taken at this time. The richest

## Constant threat of infection puts the immune force under tremendous pressure. It must be supplied with all the nutrients necessary for peak fighting performance.

eggs and fish. Eating nuts, seeds and green vegetables provides a good balance of both calcium and magnesium.

### Selenium

Selenium levels in crops and vegetables depend on the soil that they are grown in. Today, some areas of farmland have been shown to have particularly low levels of this trace mineral; consequently food grown there will be mineral-deficient, although it may look and taste perfect. Selenium is involved in antibody synthesis. Without it, an immune cell cannot efficiently copy the cells that it produces in response to a repeated infection. Like many nutrients, selenium works best in combination with a vitamin, in this case vitamin E. Rich sources of selenium are liver, shellfish, onions, garlic, wholegrains and cereals (granolas) – although a certain amount can be derived from green vegetables.

sources of iron are green vegetables, liver and wholegrain bread. It is also found in dried fruits and cereals (granolas).

### Zinc

The thymus gland requires zinc to manufacture the T-cells that fight pathogens. Zinc is also needed to aid the T-cells towards active maturity.

### Manganese

This trace mineral is required for interferon production (see page 99). The body often lacks an adequate amount of it. Its jobs are to form bone and cartilage, and control glucose metabolism. Signs that one is low in manganese include poor balance, confusion and sore knees. Good sources are wholegrain cereals (granolas), pulses (legumes), green vegetables, wheatgerm, rice bran, nuts, ginger and cloves. Factors that hinder absorption of manganese include tea, coffee, smoking and high doses of iron and zinc.

## The top ten vegetables for the immune system

When you have an infection, make sure that you eat lots of raw and lightly steamed vegetables, because they help the immune system to fight pathogens. The vegetables below are ideal, as they contain high levels of antioxidants to help combat damage by free radicals. In addition, they have strong antiviral, antibacterial and anti-fungal properties, as well as being natural antibiotics.

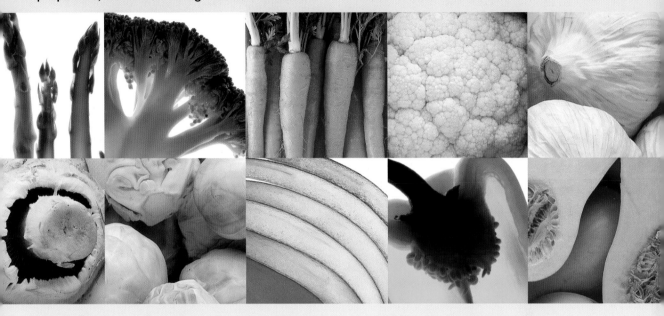

To ensure that you also get adequate carbohydrate and protein, plan meals to include lentils, wholegrain bread and brown rice, which are also good sources of minerals to boost the immune system.

### Immune Inhibitors

We have seen which nutrients boost and support the immune system, so we should also look at which nutritional and other influences hinder the workings of our vital protection force.

### Sugar

Sugar, in any form, inhibits the activity of the white cells that digest pathogens, for up to five hours after eating it. A sugary cereal (granola) at breakfast, followed by sweet snacks, soft drinks and sweet tea or coffee throughout the day, followed by an instant meal high in hidden sugars can permanently suppress your immune system. Give it up. It has no nutritional value, rots your teeth and makes you put on weight.

### Alcohol

As a simple sugar, alcohol has the same effect. Even if your immune system is in good working order, supported by a diet high in nutrients, alcohol can inhibit the beneficial activity of the immune cells. Although it is true that a glass of

## Improving immunity – power eating

**To boost your immune system, choose at least five fruits and vegetables from the list below for every day of the week.**

**Monday**
Blackcurrants, grapefruit, canteloupes, apples, carrots, beetroot, celery, kale.

**Friday**
Blueberries, peaches, papayas, cauliflower, coconut, potatoes, spinach.

**Tuesday**
Nectarines, oranges, lemons and limes, broccoli, fennel, squash and pumpkins.

**Saturday**
Strawberries, blackcurrants, cranberries, prunes, asparagus, celeriac, palm hearts, collards.

**Wednesday**
Satsumas, clementines, mangoes, Brussels sprouts, onions, tomatoes, sweet potatoes.

**Sunday**
Raspberries, cranberries, cherries, pineapple, avocados, radishes, turnips.

**Thursday**
Apricots, dates, figs, cabbage, garlic, nettles, watercress.

red wine contains important antioxidants, there is a balance to be struck. One glass of wine a day has been shown to have a positive overall effect on health (particularly the heart), but if you drink much more, the law of diminishing returns applies.

### Caffeine

Coffee, tea and fizzy drinks all contain caffeine and inhibit the absorption of vital nutrients, in addition to directly suppressing the immune system. Green tea, however, has been found to stimulate immune function, and should become a regular substitute for caffeinated black tea. Water helps to clear toxins from the body, lessening the immune system's daily struggle.

### Heavy Metals

Elements such as cadmium (in cigarettes), lead (in traffic fumes and old water pipes), aluminium (in cooking pans), uranium (in atmosphere pollution) and mercury (in amalgam fillings) are highly toxic to body tissues. Once inside the body they become deposited in soft or fatty tissues in the brain, nervous system, kidneys, liver, eyes and lungs. Due to their high free-radical activity they cause considerable damage to body cells and interfere with normal tissue function.

These elements are a constant drain on immune resources. When present in high levels these toxic minerals contribute to zinc, selenium, sulphur, iron and calcium deficiencies. Symptoms of heavy metal toxicity include headaches, migraines, poor memory, hyperactivity, nervous conditions and frequent infections. A nutrition consultant can organize a hair mineral analysis, which can be used to determine toxic levels of heavy metals. A detoxification programme can then be planned.

## Stress

Stress suppresses the production of white blood cells and can lead to the inhibition of the thymus gland. The lymphatic cells in the thymus and the lymph nodes throughout the body disintegrate, reducing the protection offered by these important parts of the immune system. For more on stress and the immune system, see pages 73–77. To learn more about the lymphatic system, see pages 120–135 on the heart and circulation.

## Bereavement

Losing someone close to you has a profound effect on the immune system. Bereavement should never be underestimated, and often old health problems will come to the forefront within a few months of a personal loss. Sometimes these conditions present themselves in an even more severe form than when they first occurred. If you are concerned, see your doctor for a check-up to ascertain whether or not the symptoms are new or a recurrence 'in sympathy'.

Bereavement does not just apply to the death of a relative or friend. There are other types of loss, such as leaving an old family home, or the breakdown of a relationship. Changing career may also have an effect on the immune system.

## Antibiotics

The immune system is closely associated with the health of the gut. The gut, or colon, contains millions of bacteria, some of which are considered 'friendly' and others which are not. The colon has a natural balance of bacteria, yet this balance is sensitive and can easily be upset, both by an excess of simple sugars and also by taking antibiotics. Doctors are nowadays trying to prescribe fewer antibiotics, because it is thought that our over-reliance on them is endangering the population's future ability to fight disease.

Many bacteria produce natural antibiotics which act against viruses, bacteria and fungal infections. If medicinal antibiotics are taken, they damage some of these friendly bacteria, along with the 'target' bacteria.

The yeast *Candida albicans*, which lives in all of us (usually quite happily), can get out of control and proliferate. In so doing, it inhibits immune action by decreasing the production of white blood cells. Frequent use of antibiotics can encourage an overgrowth of *Candida albicans*, but it can be tamed by a strict diet that excludes all sugars and includes natural antibiotics and anti-fungals such as garlic and onions.

People who have a history of antibiotic use should follow a regime that will recolonize the gut with friendly bacteria. We have seen the immune system respond very well to this treatment. We advise supplementing with 'probiotics' in the form of live, unsweetened bio yoghurt, rich in *Lactobacillus acidophilus* and *Bifidobacteria*. It should be eaten three times a week. If preferred, supplements of these probiotics are available and are more potent.

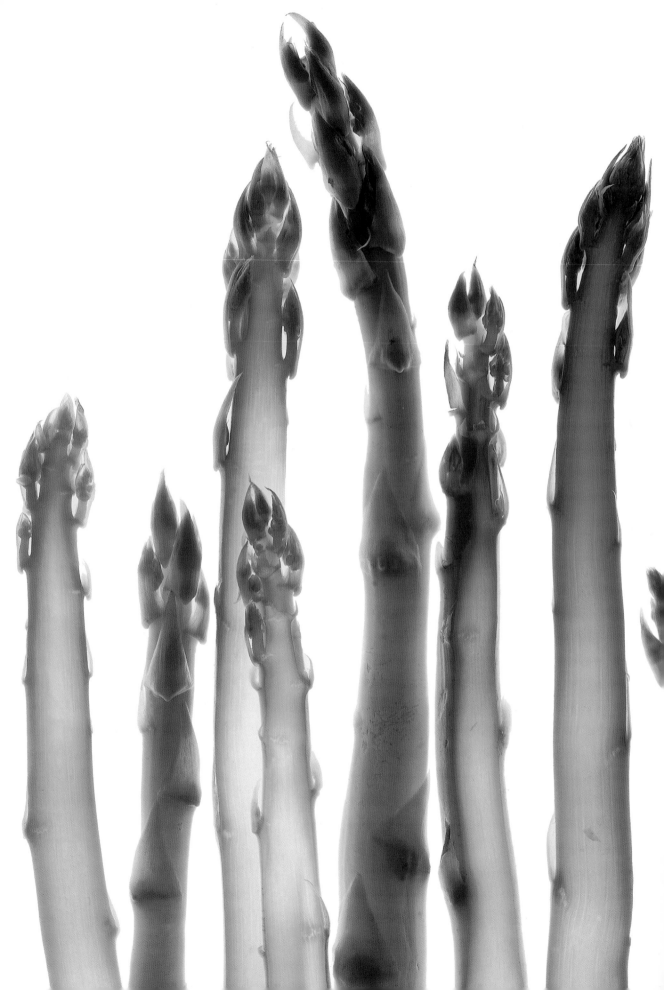

# inflammation

Inflammation is a reaction to injury, infection or an aggravating substance. Most people view an attack of inflammation, with its associated pain, swelling and redness, as unpleasant and inconvenient. However, it is actually a very positive and welcome action, necessary for the body to repair itself.

The immune system is the body's protector, swinging into action whenever it is needed. It harnesses its resources to fight off invaders such as bacteria and viruses, or to help recovery from injury and disease, or to create a reaction to an outside stimulant or aggravating factor – and for the human body, one of the most powerful of these is food. The immune system tackles the problems by providing a series of responses, inflammation being one of them.

There is a vast amount of evidence to show that our diet has a direct relationship with the immune system's ability to function well. For example, a diet rich in fruit, vegetables, essential fatty acids and wholegrains can help control the inflammation response, while a poor diet consisting predominantly of convenience foods, red meat and dairy products can promote unnecessary inflammation.

Certain foods are noted for their anti-inflammatory properties, such as strawberries and lentils. Other foods, such as tomatoes and potatoes, are thought to promote inflammation.

## Types of inflammation

There are two types of inflammation: acute and chronic. Acute inflammation occurs as the body's response to trauma (injury), irritation, infection or an allergen (ranging from chemicals to food). Chronic inflammation is a long-term problem. Contributory factors include overuse of a particular part of the body, general wear and tear and getting older.

The primary signs of acute inflammation are pain, swelling, redness and heat. These are caused by blood vessels dilating around the affected area, bringing immune mediators (substances involved in the inflammation process) to dispense with or disperse the damaged tissue or bacteria. This is the first part of the process of healing. However, if healing does not occur for any reason, chronic inflammation follows, caused by the immune system becoming either overstimulated, overactive or failing to switch off – or any combination of the three. An example of this is systemic lupus, an autoimmune condition that can affect many organs of the body (see page 117).

LEFT Asparagus is a liver tonic and helps reduce inflammation.

### The inflammation process

Inflammation is a common occurrence. Imagine what happens if we cut or knock a finger: the area becomes red and swollen, sometimes accompanied by pain, and this may lead to temporary loss of function. This reaction is the same wherever it occurs in the body, and from whatever cause – whether the injury is a physical blow, an internal stress or an irritant.

Most people react to inflammation by reaching for an anti-inflammatory painkiller. In fact, so many of us do this that non-prescription

### The three stages of inflammation

The process of inflammation is a fascinating combined effort by the skin, blood and immune cells to repair, replace and renew the damaged tissue. It takes place in three stages.

The first stage happens when the body rushes into action as soon as any part of it is affected. Immediately, the blood vessels around the injured area dilate to allow more blood to flow to the site, bringing with it the necessary nutrients and immune cells to repair and seal off the injury.

---

## Characteristics of inflammation

**Redness**

**Pain**

**Swelling**

**Heat**

**Loss of function**

### What's in a name?
In simple terms, 'itis' means 'inflamed', and is tacked on to various other words to describe problems in that area. For example, 'arthritis' describes joint inflammation ('arthro' means 'joints'). 'Dermatitis' is inflammation of the skin ('derma' means 'skin').
An 'itis' isn't the only form of inflammation. Many other conditions such as asthma, Crohn's disease (see pages 94–95) and psoriasis are also linked to the inflammatory response.

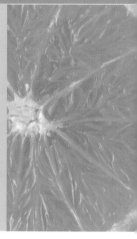

---

painkillers have become the world's biggest-selling drugs. But while inflammation may be unpleasant, it is actually a positive sign that the immune system is functioning well.

So, instead of reaching into the medicine cabinet, we should recognize that the process of inflammation is a vital function of the immune system and that when it occurs, it is only our natural defences being mobilized to deal with the injury, however small. Given a chance, the body has the ability to heal itself.

During the second stage, the immune defence team homes in on any bacteria that are present. Neutrophil cells congregate in the affected tissue, ready to engulf the bacteria completely and digest it. This amazing response, called phagocytosis, involves the cells actually changing shape – they grow tiny arms (pseudopods) that wrap around the foreign bacteria, completely overwhelming it. The cells then release chemicals that destroy the offending microbe. The cells also carry antioxidants to protect themselves from potential damage by free radicals.

It is not just the bacteria that can get eaten in the phagocytosis process. Damaged and dead cells are also removed in the same way. This leads to the third stage, when the inflamed site is made into a self-contained area, cut off from the surrounding tissue. The affected area is likely to feel sensitive, sometimes painful, and it often throbs. This forces us to rest the damaged part. Histamine is released from the immune cells (mast cells), increasing the permeability of blood vessels. This allows toxins and waste products to flow away more efficiently.

### Give me fever

The most dramatic reaction in the inflammation repertoire is fever. This occurs when there is a challenging infection that requires the immune force to be at its most potent. Fevers can be alarming, but understanding exactly what is happening can help dispel the fear. Fever creates a series of individual reactions in the body, all of which work together to fight off the cause of the fever. These responses, and their causes, are shown in the box on page 110.

Body temperature shoots up during a fever, peaking as the battle against the infection reaches its climax. But we may feel cold and shivery, ensuring that we wrap up warmly or – better still – retire to bed. The body appears to shut down. We feel weak, our senses are dulled, speech becomes difficult, food seems unappetizing and we may feel separated from the world around us. The body is telling us that it needs uninterrupted rest to repair itself. These symptoms may last for as long as three days – roughly as long as it takes the immune system to do its magical rejuvenation work.

During this shut-down time, the body is battling the invading bacteria without distraction. Bacteria survive and flourish at 98.6°F (37°C) – which is normal body temperature. While we are running a temperature, bacteria cannot thrive and their ability to reproduce is reduced. The cells that engulf them increase, called up from elsewhere in the body. As the body's temperature continues to rise, the balance of power tips in our favour: now there are fewer bacteria and an increased number of white blood cells. It is at this point that the battle has been won. The fever breaks.

### Why fever is good for you

A fever can be quite dramatic and worrying for the onlooker as well as for the person experiencing the battle raging inside the body. Modern medicine has developed methods to bring down fever; however, interrupting a fever also disrupts the natural process of defence and is often the cause of longer and repeated bouts of infection. This is frequently seen in children's ear, nose and throat infections.

This is not to say that fever should be left unchecked. In adults it is not uncommon to see a fever temperature of up to 104°F (40°C). Short periods of such high fever are usually safe, but ensure that your doctor is made aware of the condition.

**nutrition know-how**

Vitamin C can flush out toxins and lower temperature. Encourage a feverish child to sip diluted orange juice throughout the day.

**Warning**. In children, fever response is more frequent and should never be ignored. Seek medical advice if your child's high temperature is persistent or is accompanied by drowsiness, delirium, repeated vomiting or severe pain. Beware of a high fever and a skin rash that does not disappear when pressed – this could indicate meningitis and requires urgent medical help. High fever can also cause epileptic fits and may need to be controlled by cooling measures.

### Causes of inflammation

A variety of triggers lead to inflammation, including environmental, metabolic, nutritional, structural, digestive, infectious and drug-induced factors. Five substances respond to these influences: histamine, kinins, prostaglandins, leukotrienes and complement. Some are helpful, some are not. Good nutritional sources to promote or combat these five substances are listed in the chart on page 112.

### Histamine

This substance is derived from the mast cells and is made from histadine, an amino acid. Histamine has many effects on the body, some of which are involved in the immune process. It contracts the smooth muscles and encourages the dilation of blood vessels. It is released in large amounts after the skin has been damaged, as seen when a weal develops. Some people produce more histamine than others. Hayfever sufferers are typically high histamine producers.

To counter some of the effects of inflammation, it is important to reduce the production of histamine. This can be achieved without resorting to over-the-counter antihistamine preparations, simply by including some basic nutrients in your daily diet, as outlined in the chart on page 112. Taking antihistamines can have a negative effect on the body as they need to be detoxified by the liver, causing unnecessary stress. This in turn makes the liver

**The body's reaction to fever**

| Response | Reason |
|---|---|
| Raised temperature | Reduces the activity of bacteria that thrive at normal body temperature. |
| Faster breathing | Increases flow of oxygen throughout the body. |
| Faster heart rate | Pumps more blood to the affected area, to deliver essential nutrients for healing and repair. |
| Sweating | Speeds up the elimination of toxins through the skin and regulates temperature. |

less effective at detoxifying natural histamine, creating a need for antihistamines – and so the cycle continues!

### Kinins

Kinins are polypeptides ('poly' means 'many'; 'peptide' means 'protein molecule'). Like histamine, they are derived from amino acids. Unlike other parts of the immune force, however, kinins are not found circulating in the blood: they are produced only in response to tissue damage or if there is a change in body temperature, such as a fever.

The body maintains a strict balance between acidity and alkalinity and employs buffering systems to maintain it. Kinins are released into the blood if this delicate acid–alkaline balance (the pH) is altered in response to a breakdown of tissue caused by high acidity. For example, stress will encourage a highly acid state in the body, as will a high-protein diet.

### DIY test for histamine levels

To give you an indication of your histamine levels, do this simple test. Roll up your sleeve and lightly scratch the inside of your forearm from wrist to elbow. Within a minute or less, a red mark will appear where you have scratched. This is histamine being called to the site of trauma to help heal it. The greater the intensity of redness and possible swelling, the higher your histamine levels.

### Prostaglandins

Prostaglandins are very short-lived substances that act like hormones. They affect the tissue immediately around them and cause the constriction of smooth muscles. Prostaglandins are produced from essential fatty acids, which must be obtained from the diet. There are three different types of prostaglandins: Pg-1, Pg-2 and Pg-3.

Pg-1 and Pg-3 are very important to the body. They are not only anti-inflammatory, but help to reduce cholesterol, lower blood pressure and prevent blood clotting as well. They also help raise high-density lipoprotein (HDL) levels in the body to protect against heart disease.

Pg-2 is a 'bad' prostaglandin, promoting inflammation. It also raises cholesterol and blood pressure, encourages blood clotting and lowers HDL levels. Avoid Pg-2 foods, such as animal and dairy products, which are rich in saturated fats.

### Leukotrienes

Less is known about leukotrienes than some of the other mediators of inflammation. They are related to prostaglandins and generated from arachidonic acid. Leukotrienes play a role in promoting the inflammatory response, especially allergic responses.

### Complement

Complement is a protein found in the blood and is usually inactive. There are about ten different types of complement and, when activated, they improve, or complement, the immune system,

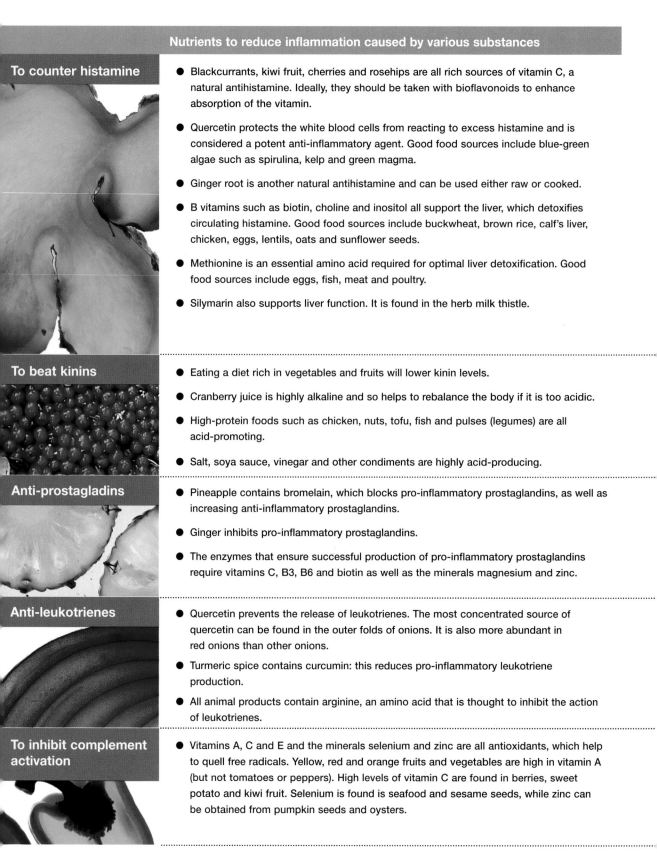

## Nutrients to reduce inflammation caused by various substances

### To counter histamine

- Blackcurrants, kiwi fruit, cherries and rosehips are all rich sources of vitamin C, a natural antihistamine. Ideally, they should be taken with bioflavonoids to enhance absorption of the vitamin.

- Quercetin protects the white blood cells from reacting to excess histamine and is considered a potent anti-inflammatory agent. Good food sources include blue-green algae such as spirulina, kelp and green magma.

- Ginger root is another natural antihistamine and can be used either raw or cooked.

- B vitamins such as biotin, choline and inositol all support the liver, which detoxifies circulating histamine. Good food sources include buckwheat, brown rice, calf's liver, chicken, eggs, lentils, oats and sunflower seeds.

- Methionine is an essential amino acid required for optimal liver detoxification. Good food sources include eggs, fish, meat and poultry.

- Silymarin also supports liver function. It is found in the herb milk thistle.

### To beat kinins

- Eating a diet rich in vegetables and fruits will lower kinin levels.

- Cranberry juice is highly alkaline and so helps to rebalance the body if it is too acidic.

- High-protein foods such as chicken, nuts, tofu, fish and pulses (legumes) are all acid-promoting.

- Salt, soya sauce, vinegar and other condiments are highly acid-producing.

### Anti-prostagladins

- Pineapple contains bromelain, which blocks pro-inflammatory prostaglandins, as well as increasing anti-inflammatory prostaglandins.

- Ginger inhibits pro-inflammatory prostaglandins.

- The enzymes that ensure successful production of pro-inflammatory prostaglandins require vitamins C, B3, B6 and biotin as well as the minerals magnesium and zinc.

### Anti-leukotrienes

- Quercetin prevents the release of leukotrienes. The most concentrated source of quercetin can be found in the outer folds of onions. It is also more abundant in red onions than other onions.

- Turmeric spice contains curcumin: this reduces pro-inflammatory leukotriene production.

- All animal products contain arginine, an amino acid that is thought to inhibit the action of leukotrienes.

### To inhibit complement activation

- Vitamins A, C and E and the minerals selenium and zinc are all antioxidants, which help to quell free radicals. Yellow, red and orange fruits and vegetables are high in vitamin A (but not tomatoes or peppers). High levels of vitamin C are found in berries, sweet potato and kiwi fruit. Selenium is found is seafood and sesame seeds, while zinc can be obtained from pumpkin seeds and oysters.

hence their name. They serve to dilate arterioles, which are tiny arteries serving the blood capillaries. Complement is also involved in the release of histamine from the mast cells, further exacerbating inflammation.

## Hyperimmunity – an immune system out of control

We can see that inflammation is a vital and efficient way for the body to repair itself, so why and how does the inflammatory process become damaging? There are four reasons why the immune system can become overstimulated.

**1** The immune system is frequently or constantly challenged.

Examples of challenges include food intolerances, environmental stresses such as toxic chemicals and pollution, infections, vaccinations, excessive alcohol, nicotine, recreational drugs, eating a diet high in saturated fats and relying too much on convenience foods.

**2** There can be an over-firing of the normal inflammatory response.

This can be attributed to deficiencies of nutrients, specifically the antioxidants and bioflavonoids responsible for neutralizing damaging free radicals.

**3** The immune system fails to shut down once the inflammation has fulfilled its function.

This leads to autoimmunity, a condition in which the body fails to recognize the difference between its own cells and foreign matter. It reaches a state of confusion (this is often precipitated by exhaustion, viruses, bacterial infections and sometimes – possibly – vaccinations), where it in effect turns against itself and attacks its own cells, rather than defending them from outside invaders.

**4** The immune force may be called into action for an inappropriate reason.

This can occur because of an overactive immune system, or as a result of damage to the cells of an organ (an example of this is rheumatoid arthritis). Foods to help combat the debilitating conditions of rheumatoid arthritis and osteoarthritis are listed in the chart on page 115.

### Endocrine involvement

The endocrine glands, such as the thyroid, pancreas and ovaries, may play a part in hyperimmunity. This happens when a person has been subjected to physical trauma, endured prolonged stress or is recovering from a long-term illness. Because the immune system is in overdrive, this puts added stress on the adrenal glands, causing hormonal imbalance. This can cause some of the body's cells to start attacking themselves. An example of this is Grave's disease and Type II (Maturity Onset) diabetes.

**nutrition know-how**
To help relieve cystitis, drink at least three glasses of unsweetened cranberry juice each day until symptoms disappear. Cranberry juice is highly alkaline, which balances the acidity of the inflamed bladder.

# allergens and inflammatory conditions

There is a strong connection between food allergies and inflammation. Typical reactions to allergens are sneezing, headaches, fluid retention and bloating. To these add inflammation, particularly of the joints, and arthritic conditions.

### Attack that stranger!

The food allergy process starts at the gut lining, which is as thin as the skin of the eyelid. Certain substances, such as vitamins and minerals, are able to cross the lining and get into the bloodstream. Sometimes, though, the gut lining allows partially digested food (which still has to be broken down completely by the digestive system) to cross over into the bloodstream. This condition is known as a leaky gut, or, to give it its proper name, increased intestinal permeability. Read more about it on page 87.

Not recognizing the food molecules in the bloodstream, the white blood cells in the immune force launch an attack. In order for the invading food type to be identified and dealt with in the future, the immune system manufactures antibodies to use against the substance, should it ever be detected in the bloodstream again. If the gut is permeable, an intolerant response is more likely to recur. This results in inflammation affecting vulnerable areas, such as the joints and cartilage.

### Food culprits

Sometimes it is a food itself that causes a direct reaction. The most common allergens in Europe are wheat, dairy products and citrus fruits. In the United States, corn is frequently used in breads and baked goods, and so it is a more common allergen than wheat. If you suspect a food allergy, work with a nutrition consultant to establish what you are sensitive to. You can then devise an eating plan that avoids these foods.

The nightshade family of vegetables contains a chemical called solanine, which arthritis sufferers can be highly sensitive to. Eliminating this family of foods from your diet can greatly reduce the frequency and severity of your arthritic symptoms. The nightshade family includes tomatoes, potatoes, aubergine, chillies and peppers.

### Inflammatory conditions
#### Osteoarthritis and rheumatoid arthritis

When people talk of arthritis, they seldom realize that there are many different forms of this debilitating joint condition. However, the two most common types are rheumatoid arthritis and osteoarthritis. There are significant differences between the two; there are also specific nutrients that will combat the diseases (see the boxes opposite). Sufferers should attempt to follow the anti-inflammatory treatment plan on page 119.

## The differences between osteoarthritis and rheumatoid arthritis

| Osteoarthritis | Rheumatoid arthritis |
| --- | --- |
| • Structural and degenerative effects.<br>• May be caused by joint strain or injury.<br>• Calcium imbalance is possible.<br>• Onset usually in middle age.<br>• Affects 90 per cent of the population.<br>• Typically attacks hips, knees and ankles.<br>• Pain or stiffness is experienced in affected joints.<br>• Occurs in a gradual, progressive manner. | • Systemic, viral or bacterial cause. A blood test will show the presence of autoimmune rheumatoid factor.<br>• Allergies, intolerances, nutrient deficiencies or free radicals may be the cause.<br>• Onset usually after the age of 30. Sometimes affects children. Afflicts three times as many women as men.<br>• Typically found in the fingers, wrists, knees and ankles.<br>• Inflammation, redness, swelling and fluid retention in the affected area.<br>• Occurs for sporadic, intermittent periods when it flares up, then goes into remission. |

## Nutrients required to combat arthritis

Follow the nutritional advice below, as well as the guidelines given in the anti-inflammatory treatment plan (see page 119).

| Osteoarthritis | Rheumatoid arthritis |
| --- | --- |
| • Chondroitin sulphate, available as a mineral supplement, for regeneration of bones, ligaments and cartilage.<br>• Calcium and magnesium for bone formation. Magnesium is essential for the reabsorption of calcium. Found in dark green leafy vegetables, cheese, nuts and seeds.<br>• Manganese, a co-factor for bone reabsorption. Found in ginger, avocados, buckwheat and spinach.<br>• Boron and silica, trace minerals found in kelp, seaweed and other sea vegetables.<br>• Vitamin D, essential for the reabsorption of calcium. Found in fish oils, or made by the body after exposure to direct sunlight. | • Essential fatty acids involved in Pg-1 and Pg-3 anti-inflammatory pathways. Found in nuts, seeds and their oils, and oily fish such as salmon and mackerel.<br>• Biotin and vitamin B3, co-factors for anti-inflammatory essential fatty acids pathways. Found in wholegrains, lentils, liver, tuna, soya and sunflower seeds.<br>• Chromium, involved in insulin-related inflammation. Found in brewer's yeast, chicken, oysters and grains.<br>• Antioxidants counteract free radicals that can cause pain and inflammation. Found in highly coloured fresh fruits and vegetables. |

### Ankylosing spondylitis

Ankylosing spondylitis is an arthritic condition, although it tends to be less well documented than other types of arthritis. Its name describes inflammation of the joints of the spine.

The disease is most common in young and middle-aged men, affecting the points at which ligaments and tendons attach to the joint bones. It usually starts where the pelvis and spine meet (the sacro-iliac joint). Classic symptoms include a rigid spine and difficulty in holding the head up when walking.

Generally, ankylosing spondylitis first affects the lower back, giving rise to symptoms of lower back pain and stiffness. In extreme cases that are left untreated, the vertebrae can fuse together, causing discomfort and pain, and severely restricting movement and mobility.

The guidelines given in the anti-inflammatory treatment plan on page 119 will certainly offer some relief and, in many cases, may help reverse the early damage of ankylosing spondylitis. However, we recommend consulting a nutrition consultant or health practitioner, as well as a physiotherapist, to devise essential exercises to help loosen the area.

### Fibromyalgia

This rheumatic disorder is characterized by chronic aching muscles with no obvious physical cause, often described by sufferers as shooting or burning pain. Fibromyalgia afflicts the lower back, neck, shoulders, thighs and upper chest, although other areas may be affected as well. The pain is often greater in the mornings. Other symptoms include stiffness, swelling, fatigue and numbness. Sleep disorders are common and patients often suffer from chronic fatigue.

The presence of 'tender points' – nine specific points, particularly sensitive to pressure – is a significant indicator of fibromyalgia. These nine points are as follows:

- Lower vertebrae of the neck.
- Second rib joint.
- Upper part of the thighbone.
- Middle of the knee joint.
- Muscles at the base of the skull.
- Neck and upper back muscles.
- Mid-back muscles.
- Side of elbow.
- Outer and upper muscles of the buttocks.

Symptoms of fibromyalgia are more common in women than men and begin in early adulthood. They become more intense with age, if left untreated. In many cases, symptoms clear up very quickly by themselves, but tend to return unless treatment is maintained. Following the guidelines given in the anti-inflammatory treatment plan (see page 119) offers assistance by reducing muscle inflammation.

### Multiple sclerosis

MS is an inflammation of the protective fatty layer surrounding the nerve cells, known as the myelin sheath. As the inflammation advances, the myelin sheath breaks down and is replaced by scar tissue, rendering the enclosed nerve ineffective. In its advanced stages, the disease can have devastating effects on a person's ability to move, speak and care for themselves.

The importance of anti-inflammatory essential fatty acids contained in fish, nuts and seeds cannot be overestimated, and pro-inflammatory foods should be completely avoided. There is much research that supports the use of dietary manipulation to relieve the painful symptoms of MS. Follow the guidelines given in the anti-inflammatory treatment plan (see page 119).

### Bronchitis and asthma

These two conditions are closely linked, and both are classified as inflammatory. Bronchitis is inflammation of the bronchial tubes; asthma describes difficulty in breathing due to inflammation of the bronchial tubes, coupled with an excessive production of mucus.

There are two categories of bronchitis. Acute bronchitis is often caused by a viral infection (usually of the respiratory tract) such as flu or the common cold. Chronic bronchitis is usually related to frequent irritation of the bronchial tubes, and can be caused by exposure to toxins, chemicals or cigarette smoke.

For asthma sufferers there are many possible villains that can set off an attack, ranging from environmental influences such as chemicals, feathers or food additives to anxiety or even low blood sugar. All can result in the muscles that surround the bronchi becoming irritated and inflamed, thereby reducing the air flow to and from the lungs and leaving the asthmatic gasping for air.

Both conditions can be greatly helped by the guidelines given in the anti-inflammatory treatment plan on page 119. While this may not address all the causes, it should help alleviate many symptoms. In all cases, seek the advice of a nutrition consultant or health practitioner to identify and eliminate the allergens.

### Lupus

Lupus is an autoimmune disease occurring when the body fails to distinguish self from non-self, and so attacks its own tissues. It can be systemic (affecting the whole body: system and organs). Some sufferers develop an unusual rash on their cheeks, which has been likened to the markings on a wolf. This gives the disease its name – 'lupus' is Latin for 'wolf'.

There are two types of lupus, both of which can differ in their severity. The less serious type, known as discoid lupus erythematosus (DLE), causes small lesions to form on the skin, leaving scars when they disappear. Systemic lupus erythematosus (SLE) is more serious, because it can affect far more than the skin. In its early stages, it is similar to arthritis, as inflammation of the joints and hands is not uncommon. A fever often accompanies these initial symptoms; many people go on to develop inflammation of the kidneys (nephritis) or other organs.

Following the guidelines given in the anti-inflammatory treatment plan (see page 119) may offer some relief, but it is essential to consult a doctor in the first instance.

### Tendinitis and bursitis

Tendinitis is inflammation of the tendons, while bursitis is the inflammation of the bursae – fluid-filled cushions that lubricate the joints, reducing friction. Both conditions usually follow some form of trauma, for example sudden pressure or strain. Repeated movements can also lead to bursitis – housemaid's knee and frozen shoulder are both examples of it.

The two conditions are both inflammatory and often difficult to tell apart. Bursitis is usually associated with painful swelling and an accumulation of fluid, while the inflammation of tendinitis is not so obvious and is less severe. Bursitis is typically characterized by a dull ache that becomes more acute with movement; a sharp pain is more common with tendinitis.

As a basis for improving both conditions, follow the guidelines given in the anti-inflammatory treatment plan opposite.

### Gout

Gout is sometimes called crystal arthritis, as it is caused by excess uric acid in the blood, tissues and urine. Uric acid is a substance that the body produces and excretes in the urine, via the kidneys.

Uric acid can crystallize into needle-shaped crystals which 'jab' at the spaces in between joints, causing pain. Gout is often found in the big toe as well as the knees and ankles. A blood test can confirm whether uric acid levels in the blood are higher than normal. Symptoms are similar to those of the other types of arthritis, in that the affected areas become painful and inflamed.

Gout used to be associated with too much high living and the consumption of rich food (because of the link between such foods and uric acid production). However, we now know that certain foods contain a substance called purine, which leads to excessive uric acid production. Purine-rich foods include meat, foods high in saturated fats, anchovies, herring, mackerel, sardines, scallops, liver, kidneys, sweetbreads and fish roe. These should all be avoided if you have a tendency to gout.

Foods low in purine include rice, millet, avocados, green vegetables, goat's milk, goat's yoghurt, eggs and non-citrus fruits. Alfalfa sprouts, celery and vitamin C all help to clear uric acid.

### Hayfever

Hayfever is an allergy to airborne particles, and it is a good example of how the inflammatory response operates in the air passages.

When a hayfever sufferer inhales airborne pollen, it causes the release of histamine as soon as the allergen makes contact with the lungs. Histamine is an inflammatory trigger (see page 110). It's not just pollen that causes hayfever: house dust mites, animal hair, feathers or chemicals can start similar reactions.

The mast cells release histamine to encourage the expulsion of the pollen or other allergen – in other words they make us sneeze! Taking an antihistamine can reduce the response, and therefore the symptoms, but, at the same time, it may suppress the immune system. As antihistamines are chemicals, they require breaking down by a liver already taxed by the presence of excess natural histamine. The cycle needs to be broken.

If you decide to take nutritional supplements, start before the hayfever season, to give your body time to accumulate immunity as well as high levels of the various nutrients.

We do of course acknowledge that many people will need to take some sort of medication. Whilst antihistamines can be effective, please be aware of the histamine/liver connection and stick to the stated dose. Many people prefer a hayfever 'jab'. This lowers histamine release and is a good way of acquiring protection for a month or so. But it also affects general immunity, leaving you more prone to colds and other infections, and is not generally recommended by the medical profession.

Dairy products, in particular cheeses, are high in saturated fat, which contributes to high levels of pro-inflammatory prostaglandins. Many people find their hayfever symptoms are greatly reduced when they cut dairy products out of their diet.

Eat foods that are rich in the anti-inflammatory vitamins A, B and C, calcium, bioflavonoids, quercetin, methionine and co-enzyme Q10.

## Your natural anti-inflammatory treatment plan

- Avoid foods such as citrus fruits, wheat, eggs, shellfish, dairy products and chocolate. Much allergy-related inflammation is triggered by these foods.

- Don't eat foods from the nightshade family, which includes potatoes, tomatoes, peppers, aubergines (eggplants), Cape gooseberries (physalis), rhubarb and courgettes (zucchini).

- Choose foods rich in vitamin A, found in red and yellow fruits and vegetables such as plums, peaches, pumpkins, squash and beetroot.

- Pick foods rich in vitamin C, such as strawberries, kiwi fruit and sweet potatoes.

- Eat foods containing bioflavonoids, which support vitamin C production. They are found in yellow and green vegetables such as squash, broccoli and kale, and dark berries such as blackcurrants.

- Avocados, sesame seeds, pumpkin seeds and sunflower seeds are rich in vitamin E, which is helpful for calming inflammation.

- Quercetin is a potent anti-inflammatory because it slows down histamine release. Quercetin is found in onions and kelp.

- Methionine is an amino acid found in protein foods. It binds to the excess histamine, making reactions less severe. Grade-A protein foods include tuna, mackerel, herring, sardines, salmon, chicken and tofu.

- Bromelain is one of the most powerful anti-inflammatories, and is found in pineapples and nuts.

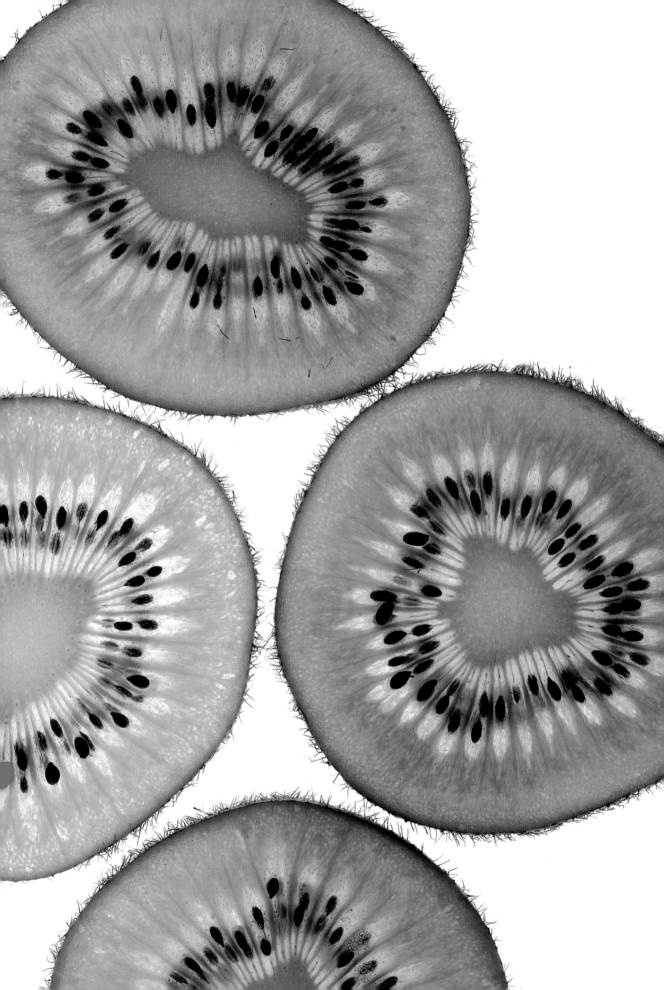

# the heart and circulation

Research shows that the heart is capable of recovering from damage. As heart disease is one of the most common causes of death, making changes to diet and lifestyle are worthwhile. This hard-working muscle pumps around 17,600 pints (10,000 litres) of blood around the body every day.

The early stages of arterial disease carry few symptoms. In fact, most sufferers are unaware of any problems until they experience a heart attack or a stroke. Despite this, heart disease is the second biggest cause of death in the United Kingdom, accounting for nearly 170,000 deaths each year. Approximately one in three men and one in four women die from this disease. In the United States, heart disease accounts for more than one million deaths annually. And most heart problems can be avoided – or improved significantly – through diet.

The driving force of the cardiovascular system is the heart, which pumps blood around the body through an intricate series of veins and arteries. Essentially, the heart is a powerful muscle which requires nutrients of its own to carry out its job. The blood acts as a carrier, delivering fresh oxygen (and nutrients) to all the tissues, muscles and cells throughout the body.

Branching off the larger vessels of the heart are tiny blood capillaries that diffuse oxygen into the cells and remove waste products. The blood takes the waste products and disposes of them through the kidneys, liver and lungs. Back in the lungs, the blood is refreshed with oxygen and the cycle takes place all over again.

The veins and arteries that service the heart have different functions. Arteries transport newly oxygenated blood away from the heart; veins transport deoxygenated blood towards the heart. It may be easier to understand this if we imagine the blood as a conveyor belt running through the body, on to which gases are loaded, delivered, reloaded and exchanged at the appropriate point.

## The lymphatic system

The lymphatic system is a completely closed and separate system from that of the arteries and veins, but it is an integral part of the circulation system. The fluid that runs through its arterial-type system, with one-way valves to prevent backflow, is called lymph. Its purpose is to carry away toxins from the arteries and veins. The lymphatic system is actually part of the immune system, filtering potentially harmful substances and

LEFT Vitamin C is a potent guard against heart disease. Kiwi fruit is full of this vital nutrient.

detoxifying them. The lymph passes through lymph glands, which are large collecting areas that trap circulating bacteria and viruses and prevent them from running riot throughout the body. The glands contain and form lymphocytes, a type of white blood cell. The T-lymphocytes are involved in attacking invading organisms. The lymph glands are found all over

atherosclerosis (see page 127), which raises blood pressure. Small particles of the 'plaster' can become dislodged and travel through the blood, only to get stuck and totally block the diameter of a blood vessel further downstream. This can prevent blood and oxygen from reaching either the heart (causing a heart attack) or the brain (causing a stroke).

## Just ten years after stopping smoking, the likelihood of cardiovascular complications will have reduced to almost the same as that of someone who has never smoked.

the body: under the arms, in the groin and under the jawbone in particular. This explains the 'swollen glands' we experience when we have a bacterial infection – it is the immune system dealing with the infection.

### Factors contributing to heart disease

Having examined how the heart works, let's look at the factors that can contribute to coronary heart disease.

Artery, vein and capillary walls are at risk of damage as the blood travels at remarkable speeds, and just like a river erodes its banks, so the blood vessels are at constant risk of degeneration. Once damaged the body sets about a repair job, so that blood does not escape into surrounding body tissue. Tiny holes and tears are plastered up with blood components such as sticky fatty substances, minerals such as calcium and proteins including fibrinogen. Patching up the holes has the effect of furring-up or narrowing the inside diameter of blood vessels, a process called

Strong, flexible blood vessel walls are imperative for a healthy and protected circulatory system. Vitamin C found in citrus fruits, kiwi fruit, parsley, watercress and potatoes, and sulphur found in fish, meat, cabbage, onions and garlic are required for the collagen formation used in blood vessel walls.

### Gender

Men suffer more coronary heart disease than women. As yet, we do not know why this is. However, once women reach the menopause and no longer have the protective female hormone oestrogen, their rate of disease roughly matches that of men.

### Excess weight

Being overweight is known to increase blood pressure and affect the sensitive ratio of 'bad' cholesterol (low-density lipoproteins, or LDL) to 'good' cholesterol (high-density lipoproteins, or HDL). Obese people are often unable to exercise, further raising their risk of being affected by cardiovascular complications. Carrying excess weight around puts a strain on all the body organs, especially the heart, which has to pump harder. As fat accumulates in the body, it also increases in the arteries.

### Age

The risk of coronary heart disease rises with age, because damage to the arteries accumulates over the years and blood pressure rises accordingly, presenting a risk factor.

### Trans fats intake

A high intake of trans fats, derived from saturated fats found in animal products, increases the risk of coronary heart disease. Many products, such as margarine, cakes and biscuits, contain it. In the blood, the trans fats are converted to triglycerides, a high level of which can increase cardiovascular problems, and raise cholesterol levels.

### Smoking

Smoking increases the occurrence of free radicals, using up the body's supply of vitamin C, thereby increasing the risk of arteriosclerosis. It also introduces nicotine and carbon monoxide into the blood. Nicotine constricts the blood vessels, exacerbating the risk of thrombosis or heart attack. Carbon monoxide encourages blood clotting and reduces oxygen levels in body tissues and muscles, including the heart muscle. Regular cigarette smoking is thought to increase the risk of cardiovascular disease by at least 100 per cent. Both cigarette and cigar smokers are at risk of oral cancers, whether or not they inhale.

The body's remarkable ability to recover is underlined in the risk factors for smoking. Just ten years after stopping smoking, the likelihood of cardiovascular complications will have reduced to almost the same as that of someone who has never smoked. This means that it is always worth giving up smoking, whatever your age and no matter how long you have smoked.

### Hypertension

If the flow of blood through the circulatory system is impeded, the internal circumference of the arteries is reduced. This is one of the main reasons for high blood pressure. Taking a blood-pressure reading gives a clue about the condition of the intima (the internal layers of the arteries and veins). A high reading may indicate the presence of atherosclerosis.

### Lack of exercise

A lack of regular exercise has been proved to have a detrimental effect on the cardiovascular system. Take regular aerobic exercise to work all muscles, including the heart muscle itself, increasing its capacity and endurance. As the heart beats harder, blood flows faster, ensuring better delivery of nutrients and oxygen to every part of the body, as well as more efficient removal of waste by the blood. Exercise also increases levels of the HDL 'good' cholesterol.

**nutrition know-how**

The omega-3 essential fatty acids found in oily fish and sunflower and pumpkin seeds reduce blood coagulation. Eating a handful of these valuable seeds every day, and a portion of fish 3–4 times per week, is recommended.

## Heart helpers

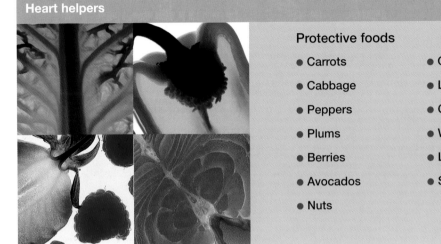

### Protective foods

- Carrots
- Cabbage
- Peppers
- Plums
- Berries
- Avocados
- Nuts

- Oily fish
- Liver
- Garlic
- Wholegrains
- Lentils
- Spinach

### Alcohol

Apart from the fact that excessive alcohol leads to weight gain and raised blood pressure, alcohol also encourages platelets in the blood to become stickier. This makes the blood thicker, impeding its passage through the blood vessels.

However, red wine contains a substance called quinone, an antioxidant that can help to reduce cholesterol and prevent plaque deposits. Two or three glasses a week are thought to be beneficial, but more than this can be harmful. Alcohol also encourages the excretion of magnesium, and this mineral is essential for a healthy heart.

### Diabetes

The condition known as Type II diabetes mellitus (see page 10) carries with it the risk of hypertension. The diabetic's body produces large quantities of insulin, yet the circulating sugar in the blood does not respond to it, so the smallest blood vessels can become coated in sugar (glycosolated). This makes the risk of heart disease up to ten times greater for those who suffer from this type of diabetes.

### Family history

It is thought that 25 per cent of the population has an increased risk of heart attacks due to genetic disposition. This is believed to be linked to arterial deterioration which occurs in people not expected to be at high risk (they have never smoked, take regular exercise, have good diets, maintain their correct weight and have normal blood pressure). Generally, if there is a family history of heart disease, extra care needs to be taken with diet and lifestyle.

A minority of people, estimated to be roughly 1 in 500, suffers from a condition known as familial hypercholesterolaemia. This genetic error causes unusually high levels of cholesterol to circulate in the blood. Families with hypercholesterolaemia have to be particularly vigilant about their diet (making sure they avoid all saturated fats) and lifestyle choices.

### Homocysteine

Recent research has confirmed the involvement of another possible genetic factor in heart disease. Homocysteine is a protein metabolite which, like all other products of metabolism, needs to be cleared from the body efficiently. In some people it can build up, to detrimental effect.

It has been found that certain vitamins, namely B6 and B12, are often deficient in those with high homocysteine levels in the blood. Taking a supplement of these vitamins, together with the amino acid methionine, can help clear pathways, preventing long-term damage.

Research has been going on in this area for over 30 years, but the medical profession has taken a long time to recognize that this genetic factor may play an even larger part in the development of heart disease than cholesterol. Tests to measure homocysteine levels are now readily available, and form part of a thorough diagnostic cardiovascular screening.

### Stress

Stress is an unavoidable part of life. Continued stress encourages the body to release adrenaline, which is responsible for making the blood thicker and stickier. This is part of the 'fight or flight' syndrome (see pages 71–73), when the body responds to danger or challenge. Excess adrenaline in the blood is eventually converted into a substance called adrenochrome. This has free radical properties that can lead to the first stage of atherosclerosis, because the intima (internal layers) of the arteries are damaged.

Continued stress stimulates the breakdown of bone, releasing stores of calcium into the blood. This encourages calcification of the arteries, as well as potentially increasing the risk of osteoporosis (for more on this condition, see page 75). Stress also encourages the excretion of magnesium (see pages 75–76). The balance of these two essential minerals is crucial to the health of smooth muscle tissue found in the heart itself: calcium precipitates its contraction and magnesium its relaxation.

### Salt

In the body, salt (sodium) and potassium are delicately balanced in all cells. Together, they are responsible for maintaining water levels in the cells, and the intake/output of nutrients and waste matter. If there is additional salt coming into the body through the diet, this balance is disturbed, resulting in increased blood pressure.

Salt occurs naturally in food. For example, raw broccoli contains approximately 0.25 per cent sodium and carrots contain approximately 0.3 per cent. While this may not sound like much, someone eating just three portions of vegetables a day is easily getting enough sodium for the body.

Eating any processed food – whether it is a snack, a ready meal, or even canned vegetables – will cause an excessive amount of sodium to be taken in by the body. Food manufacturers use a lot of salt in their products because it is cheap and provides some flavour. If you feel that you can't taste your food and have to put salt on it, then you may be deficient in zinc. Check this for yourself by taking the zinc test on page 80.

To get the best out of your taste buds, you need adequate amounts of zinc. Talk to your nutrition consultant about taking a zinc supplement, as quantities of this mineral should not exceed 45 mg per day.

### The cholesterol connection

Cholesterol used to be much feared. Less than 20 years ago it was thought to be the major cause of heart disease. Although it is certainly a contributory factor, it is important to remember that our bodies actually need and manufacture cholesterol every day for vital functions.

Cholesterol is a naturally occurring substance in the body, produced by the liver in varying quantities (but usually less than 3 g per day). It is used in cell membranes and for the formation of sex and stress hormones; it is required for the synthesis of vitamin D, and in the nervous system it is a constituent of the myelin sheath, the protective covering on all nerves. Usually, any excess cholesterol in the body binds with fibre and is excreted via the bowels. However, if large amounts accumulate, they can cause the formation of gallstones, or may be stored as fat in cellulite, or be seen as small white or yellowish spots below the eyes.

There are two types of cholesterol: high-density lipoprotein (HDL) and low-density lipoprotein (LDL). The two balance each other. The HDL removes cholesterol from vulnerable areas, taking it back to the liver for recycling and disposal, while the LDL does the opposite – it delivers cholesterol throughout the body to where it is required. Both are carried in the blood. The ratio between the two should ideally be 2:1 in favour of the HDL. However, many of us have raised levels of LDL and reduced HDL, upsetting the ideal balance and allowing the potentially harmful cholesterol to build up in the body.

The facts are clear – LDL cholesterol levels are increased by a high intake of saturated fats. These fats are found in red meat, full-fat dairy products and fried foods. The more of these foods that we eat, the higher our LDL cholesterol levels are likely to be. To counterbalance this, foods rich in omega-6 (nuts and seeds) and in particular omega-3 (oily fish and flax oil) essential fatty acids are known to raise protective HDL levels.

However, if the amount of cholesterol taken in from dietary sources is too high, a healthy body will reduce the amount it produces accordingly. Cholesterol can also build up if there is too much in the blood, or it is not excreted because of a lack of fibre in the diet.

### Heart diseases

#### Arteriosclerosis

In this condition, the arteries thicken due to calcium salts from the blood being deposited in the arteries, or because of the deterioration of the connective tissue of the heart. This thickening leads to a loss of elasticity, which in turn reduces the flexibility of the blood vessels. Although often considered to be part of the normal process of ageing, many factors can contribute to increased, and possibly unnecessary, incidence of arteriosclerosis.

**nutrition know-how**

The perfect meal for heart health would include some fish, at least two types of vegetables and a little wholegrain brown rice. This provides high levels of protein, EPA, antioxidants, B-complex vitamins, calcium, zinc and magnesium.

The condition is very common, and together with atherosclerosis (see below), it is one of the primary causes of heart attacks and strokes. Nutrition plays a powerful role in avoiding these conditions.

### Atherosclerosis

The arteries are lined with a layer of smooth tissue, known as the intima, which can become coated in a plaque not unlike the one that builds up on teeth. In time, this plaque forms a lesion of irregular cells.

In an attempt to repair the lesion damage, more smooth muscle cells are produced. But the damaged cells do not divide correctly and substances constantly flowing past in the blood, such as LDL cholesterol, calcium and platelets, attach to this mass, making it grow larger and narrowing the space available for the blood to pass through.

In time, the internal circumference of the artery is reduced as the damaged area grows. Other lesions that have broken away further along the flow can then become lodged in the narrowed artery, causing a blockage.

Depending on where the blockage actually occurs, the resulting starvation of oxygen will either cause a heart attack (if it is in the circulation around the heart) or a stroke (if it is nearer the brain).

There has been much research into how the arteries become damaged in the first place, creating the need for repair, and it is thought that free radicals play a major role. This means that there is a need for antioxidants, which protect the intima. Vitamin C in particular is required for maintaining the integrity of the arterial wall and research has shown that it can effect repair.

### Angina pectoris

Angina simply means 'pain', and 'pectoris' means 'in the chest': angina pectoris is chest pain. This is a common condition. It results from what is known as 'ischemia', which is a reduced blood flow to a part of the body. If blood flow is limited, the area suffers a reduction in oxygen and nutrient supply. This has the effect of compromising the capacity of the cells without actually destroying them. The heart has its own blood supply to keep it working. When ischemia occurs, the heart continues to pump as hard as usual, but it is not receiving enough oxygen and nutrients to support its exertions.

Angina comes on after a period of this unsupported exertion, perhaps following exercise or climbing the stairs. Symptoms include pain in the middle of the chest, arms and jaw, dizziness and weakness.

### Heart attack (myocardial infarction)

A heart attack happens when the blood supply to the heart is cut off by a blockage, either in the blood vessels leading to the heart, or in the circulation within the heart muscle itself. As we know, heart attacks can be fatal. However, many people do survive them, because the severity of the attack depends on where in the heart the blockage has occurred. If someone survives a heart attack, areas of the heart tissue will have died and are replaced by scar tissue. Scar tissue is not flexible, leading to a reduction in the heart's ability to function normally. Imagine trying to blow up a balloon where one part of it is covered in sticky tape – that part remains solid and inflexible, reducing the amount of air that the balloon can take. Apply this to the heart, and it's obvious that it will not have the capacity to pump as much blood as before. There are three stages in the build-up to a heart attack. They are as follows:

Step 1 – A combination of high blood pressure and accumulated free-radical damage (which has not been balanced out by a sufficient intake of antioxidants) is thought to damage the intima. A lesion forms.

Step 2 – Plaque collects at the damaged site, and other substances in the blood attach themselves to it. The plaque grows, causing an increase in blood pressure. The body is always vigilant and aware of damage, and having sensed a problem, it will send more white blood cells to the affected area. These cells simply add to the plaque. More free radicals are produced through a series of events, causing further damage, and so the cycle starts again.

Step 3 – A piece of the plaque breaks away under the pressure of the blood rushing past, and blocks an artery. Part of the heart is deprived of its oxygen, and a heart attack then occurs.

### Stroke

Stroke is the third most common cause of death in the UK. It affects many people in their 40s and 50s, as well as those who are older. Simply put, a stroke is similar to a heart attack, except that the brain is the target organ. The arteries carrying oxygen and vital nutrients to the brain become impeded by atherosclerosis or arteriosclerosis (or both), causing arterial narrowing and the risk of blockage. If the brain is starved of oxygen for more than a couple of minutes, corresponding brain damage will inevitably occur.

Various parts of the body's motor co-ordination will be affected, depending on which artery is involved, and which parts of the brain are damaged. For some, the effects are relatively minor, such as the inability to move a limb; whilst for others, the effects are devastating, causing total paralysis to one side of the body or, at worst, bringing immediate death. For the fortunate ones, partial or even total recovery is possible, although this can take months or even years because the affected nerve transmission is slow to repair.

The causative factors are many – genetic susceptibility, high-fat diets, being overweight or obese, high blood pressure, raised HDL cholesterol levels, lack of exercise, a sedentary lifestyle and the ageing process.

Nutritional approaches for avoiding stroke include a diet low in saturated fats, regular consumption of oily fish to reduce the

## nutrition know-how

Cooking with turmeric can help reduce cholesterol levels as it contains curcuminoid, a substance shown to have a positive effect on 'bad' cholesterol. Indian cooking includes many soluble fibres and vegetables in its spicy curries, which balance the saturated fats of the chicken, lamb and beef dishes.

accumulation of arterial cholesterol and a high intake of fibre. Vitamin E is essential to reduce platelet aggregation and lower blood pressure, as well as neutralizing free-radical damage.

## High blood pressure

There are several causes for high blood pressure. One of the most common today is stress, which raises circulating cortisol levels (see pages 74–75 on stress), causing the arteries to constrict and blood pressure to rise, as in the 'fight or flight' syndrome. Whilst this is appropriate on occasion, in situations where the body needs to be on the alert, the more commonplace scenario of continual 'executive stress' is both long-term

and replace animal proteins with other sources such as fish, nuts and seeds.

Fresh vegetables and fruit provide necessary antioxidants and should form a large part of the day's meals. If you usually sip stimulant drinks throughout the day, replace them with herbal teas, plenty of mineral water and fruit or vegetable juices. Beans and legumes contain soluble fibres that also have cholesterol-lowering properties. They are an excellent source of vegetable protein, and should be enjoyed frequently, replacing some of the meals based on animal protein. Black-eyed beans, kidney beans and borlotti beans make a delicious as well as a nutritious contribution to

# The arteries and veins serving the heart must remain flexible and free of blockages, and this is where good nutrition is vital.

and damaging. Other contributors to high blood pressure include smoking, regular alcohol consumption, an excess of salt, high intake of animal (saturated) fats and obesity. Stimulants such as coffee, tea and alcohol are major culprits.

The answer to beating high blood pressure is a change of lifestyle, rather than attempting a quick fix (like short-term measures to get you through an insurance medical). High blood pressure is one of the body's warning signs: don't ignore it. Start cutting out processed foods, smoked products and convenience foods, and increase eating lean proteins. Do not add salt to your cooking or to meals – this can upset the delicate balance of the sodium–potassium pump (see pages 141–142). There is already sufficient salt present in all foods. Eat fewer dairy foods,

recipes. Regular exercise is essential for lowering high blood pressure, but if you have not exercised for some time, it should be undertaken with care. Seek the advice of your medical practitioner to establish the most suitable form for you.

## Varicose veins

Whilst a hereditary factor is often implicated in the occurrence of varicose veins, there are other considerations to be taken into account, in which diet and lifestyle play a large part. Carrying excess weight will burden the veins in the pelvis and legs, placing extra strain on the valves that encourage the regular flow of blood back up towards the heart. In addition, the walls of the veins may become damaged because of high pressure and sluggish lymphatic drainage, which leads to the bulging blue veins associated with this condition. Jobs that involve standing up all day, such as hairdressing, tend to increase the likelihood of varicose veins, as gravity also places a burden on the valves. For the same reason, it is important to avoid crossing the legs when sitting, to ensure unimpeded blood flow.

From a nutritional perspective, it is important to include plenty of vitamin C and bioflavonoids in your meals. Vitamin C is excellent for protecting the intima layer and the walls of veins and arteries throughout the body. Bioflavonoids also strengthen the walls, preventing them from weakness and bulging. Both vitamin C and bioflavonoids are found in rich supply in dark red berry fruits and citrus fruits, especially grapefruit. In the winter months, when cherries and blackcurrants are unavailable, you can substitute the tinned variety, because their nutrient content is well preserved by this method of storage.

### Poor circulation

If you often get cold hands and feet, it's likely that you suffer from poor circulation, the causes of which are similar to those for varicose veins. A slow-moving lymphatic system, the over-consumption of saturated fats (such as those found in animal produce), smoking and a high salt intake can all contribute to sluggish circulation, as can lack of exercise.

Stopping smoking is essential. Increasing fibre in the diet, to remove saturated fats and cholesterol, is important. Make vegetables and legumes a main part of meals. Fruits containing vitamin C and bioflavonoids, such as strawberries, raspberries, kiwi fruit, citrus fruits, currants and berries, will help to improve the condition.

### Thrombosis

A thrombosis occurs when a blood clot (thrombus) forms within an enclosed, undamaged blood vessel. Blood clotting usually occurs as a natural part of the healing process after an injury has damaged skin, organs or body tissue, in order to prevent excessive loss of blood. Blood should not clot, however, if there has been no damage.

If a clot builds up in an artery leading to the heart (known as a coronary thrombosis), it will prevent the essential flow of blood carrying oxygen and nutrients, and cause a heart attack. Likewise, a thrombus in the arteries leading to the brain is a common cause of stroke. A thrombus can form anywhere in the body, such as in the legs, intestines, eyes or kidneys, giving rise to extreme pain and loss of function. If a fragment of a thrombus breaks off (called an embolus), the results can be equally damaging, as it may cause a blockage in another part of the body (an embolism).

The causes of both thrombosis and embolism are the same as for atherosclerosis. In each case, the delicate balance of blood-clotting mechanisms has been disrupted by smoking, a high intake of saturated fats, excessive amounts of sugar and sweetened foods, obesity or lack of exercise. Dietary factors are extremely important in regaining health – the reduction of red meats, sugars, processed and fast foods will allow the arterial damage to repair itself. Vitamin C is vital for arterial repair, as is vitamin E, which is the most important antioxidant for neutralizing damage to the intima of the blood vessels by cholesterol and saturated fats.

## Essentials for a healthy heart

Maintaining the health of your heart is crucial if you want to lead a long, healthy and happy life. If you look after your heart, you will be able to maintain fitness levels and keep busy and active into old age. So, take note of the following factors.

- Make sure your diet is low in saturated fats. Avoid foods high in sugars or refined carbohydrates.

- Take regular exercise, such as walking, swimming or cycling.

- Eat foods rich in vitamin C, vitamin E, beta-carotene, essential fatty acids, zinc and selenium.

- Do not smoke.

- Do not drink more than the recommended amount of alcohol. (7–10 units of alcohol a week for men and women should be the maximum.)

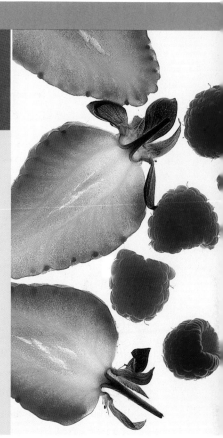

Essential fatty acids from the omega-3 group are vital for balancing the blood-clotting mechanisms throughout the circulatory system.

Most people in the West tend to have a higher intake of omega-6 essential fatty acids, because of the foods commonly eaten. This imbalance can be redressed in favour of the omega-3 group by increasing the amount of oily fish in the diet, such as salmon, tuna, mackerel, herring and sardines. Regular consumption of flaxseeds (linseeds), pumpkin and sunflower seeds has the same beneficial effect.

### Blood clotting

The phenomenon of blood clotting is a familiar one – when we suffer a cut, the blood that oozes out of the wound soon thickens and forms a clot, stopping the escape of the precious fluid. This forms the initial stage of repair to the injured site. Two components of the blood are responsible for clotting. The blood platelets work in conjunction with a protein called fibrin. The platelets coagulate into a mass that the fibrin can fasten on to. Fibrin is converted from fibrinogen. It is possible for a doctor to measure fibrinogen levels: a high level indicates that the patient is at risk from heart disease.

In heart disease, platelets can clump together in the bloodstream. Studies have shown that people who have just had a heart attack, or who are at high risk of one, have higher levels of platelet aggregation in the blood.

### Heart nutrition

Having now examined some of the factors involved in cardiovascular disease, it should be clear why certain nutrients and foods are recommended for a healthy heart. The Fighting Five – vitamins A, C, E and the minerals selenium and zinc – are essential heart nutrients. The antioxidant properties of these five nutrients help to quash the free radicals that are produced

such as antacids and analgesics (pain killers), the liver will not be able to emulsify and break down the dietary fats, causing a build-up of cholesterol and other lipids.

Regular consumption of dairy foods, animal meats and rich foods slows down the digestion, which results in constipation and toxins being re-absorbed into the bloodstream.

## Regular aerobic exercise is important for clearing excess cholesterol and working the heart muscle. Include walking, cycling or swimming in your weekly repertoire to invigorate the circulation.

as a natural by-product of metabolism (see page 140) – oxidative damage, as we have seen, plays a major part in arterial damage. Even more free radicals are produced as a result of smoking, pollution and eating fried foods.

### The importance of digestion

A healthy digestive system is vital to absorb the nutrients required for optimum heart function.

'Heartburn', or indigestion, is often an early indication of the type of daily stress the heart has to cope with. Insufficient hydrochloric acid in the stomach will not allow proteins to be broken down, causing a burning sensation and an 'over-full' feeling. This can occur after an evening meal, when going to bed soon after eating places extra strain on the digestive system.

If the liver is already overloaded by frequent drinking, over-the-counter or prescription drugs

In order to improve digestion generally and benefit from the following heart nutrients, observe the following guidelines:

● Eat small meals regularly throughout the day.
● Aid proper digestion by chewing your food well.
● Ensure that at least five to seven portions of fruits and vegetables are consumed every day to increase the fibre content, removing excess cholesterol from the digestive tract.
● Drink only small amounts of fluids at meal times to prevent the digestive enzymes from being diluted.
● Eat plenty of foods that help liver function. These include asparagus, artichokes and beetroot.
● Include raw vegetable juices regularly in your diet, as they contain high levels of nutrients.
● Eat a light evening meal.

On the next few pages we look at each antioxidant individually, as well as discussing some other beneficial nutrients for the heart.

### ● Vitamin A

Vitamin A comes in two forms, and it is beta-carotene that is most important as an antioxidant. Beta-carotene also strengthens blood capillaries.

*Good sources: red, yellow and orange fruits and vegetables such as peaches, peppers, plums and berries.*

### ● Vitamin C

Vitamin C is perhaps one of the most powerful nutrients for combating cardiovascular disease. It has been shown to lower cholesterol levels by reducing LDL and increasing HDL. It helps regulate blood pressure by thinning the blood and has powerful antioxidant properties.

*Good sources: strawberries, kiwi fruit, potatoes and oranges.*

### ● Vitamin E

Vitamin E has many benefits for the cardiovascular system. It strengthens blood vessels, reduces blood viscosity (stickiness), regulates the heartbeat and increases levels of HDL while at the same time protecting LDL from harmful free radicals.

Many nutrients work more efficiently in conjunction with another. Vitamin E is understood to work especially well with selenium to protect the cardiovascular system.

*Warning:* Take care with vitamin E if you are on heart medication (such as an anti-coagulant, for example Warfarin). If you are taking this type of drug, always check with your doctor before taking vitamin E supplements. (In such cases, high doses – 800 iµ daily – are not recommended. Your doctor may advise you to take small doses at first, building up to 400 iµ a day over three months.)

*Good sources: wheatgerm oil, oily fish such as salmon and mackerel, nut oils, eggs, green vegetables and avocados.*

### ● Selenium

The body makes antioxidant compounds and enzymes to combat naturally occurring free radicals. One of these antioxidant enzymes is called glutathione peroxidase, and the body requires selenium for its production. Selenium is a mineral found in the soil.

Modern farming pressures require farmers to grow crops year after year in the same fields, which greatly depletes the selenium content of the land. Vegetables grown in soil that is rich in the mineral will have a higher selenium content than those grown in a more impoverished soil. Even eggs have a variable selenium content: if chickens eat feed that is high in selenium, their eggs will contain a high level of it.

*Good sources: liver, fish, seafood, sesame seeds, wholegrains, onions and garlic.*

### ● Zinc

Zinc is required for the synthesis of the natural antioxidant super oxide dismutase (SOD). To test your own levels of this important nutrient, turn to the test on page 80.

*Good sources: shellfish, wholegrains such as rye and buckwheat, almonds and cashews.*

● **Magnesium**

The balance of potassium and sodium in the body affects blood pressure, and this balance is regulated by magnesium. For this reason, magnesium deficiency can cause an increase in blood pressure.

Magnesium works with calcium in all muscles and is responsible for their ability to relax. As the heart muscle contracts and relaxes more than any other in the body, a lack of magnesium can affect the rhythmic action of the heart and lead to arrhythmia (irregular heartbeat). Surgeons often prescribe magnesium supplements after heart bypass operations.

If you eat a lot of refined sugars and alcohol, it encourages the excretion of magnesium, so cut down on these.

*Good sources: fish, seafood, lentils, soya beans, nuts, seeds, dried fruits and green leafy vegetables.*

● **Co-enzyme Q10**

This remarkable nutrient is involved in energy production at a cellular level. Each cell has a tiny power plant in it – the mitochondria – which burns fuel to make energy. The more physical exertion we undertake, the greater the number of mitochondria we have, because they multiply according to the body's requirements. As the hardest-working muscle in the body, the heart has one of the highest numbers of mitochondria. Therefore, ensuring high levels of co-enzyme Q10 assists the heart muscle in its constant work. It is interesting to note that co-enzyme Q10 can be made in the body

from other enzymes, but our ability to do this declines as we age. We can also get co-enzyme Q-10 directly from the food that we eat. In Japan it is common to take supplements, and this is becoming more widespread in the West.

*Good sources: sardines, mackerel, green beans and spinach.*

● **B vitamins**

The B group of vitamins are all essential for energy production. However, vitamins B3, B5 and B6 are extra-important for preventing cardiovascular disease.

● **B3**

Vitamin B3 comes in two forms: niacin and niacinamide. Niacin can cause a flushing sensation because it dilates blood vessels. It is for precisely this reason that it is so useful in protecting the cardiovascular system – dilating blood vessels helps keep blood pressure down.

Both types of vitamin B3 reduce LDL and raise HDL, as well as being effective in the treatment of diabetes, a condition which carries with it a high risk of cardiovascular disease (see page 122).

*Good sources: green leafy vegetables, such as kale, spinach and cabbage, and wholegrains including millet and rye.*

● **B5**

Vitamin B5, or pantothenic acid, can increase HDL levels, improving the ratio between the good and bad cholesterols. It is also involved in reducing stress.

*Good sources: firm green vegetables, such as broccoli and Brussels sprouts, as well as barley and wholegrain brown rice.*

### B6

Vitamin B6, or pyroxidine, together with vitamin B12, is essential for preventing the build-up of homocysteine, which can be partly responsible for the 'furring up' of the arteries.

*Good sources: wholegrains, liver, kidneys, eggs, vegetables including cabbage, watercress and parsley.*

### Oils and fats

One type of oil, known as eicosapentaeoic acid (EPA), has been shown to lower blood pressure, reduce LDL and raise HDL and lessen the adhesion of platelets, and therefore the stickiness of the blood.

As EPA is an oil, it has double bonds in its chemical structure and these double bonds are vulnerable to free radicals. Always balance oils and fats with antioxidants.

Another type of fat, saturated fat, should be avoided because it can encourage raised LDL and blood triglycerides, and also contribute to the 'clogging' of arteries, in conditions such as arteriosclerosis and atherosclerosis.

*Good sources: nuts, seeds, fish (especially cold-water fish such as mackerel, salmon, haddock and sardines), blue green algae such as spirulina or chlorella. Health authorities suggest that we should all eat oily fish at least three times a week, but we suggest that you try to eat it five times a week and also have a handful of nuts every day.*

### Fibre

Fibre is essential for maintaining healthy heart function, as it is required for the removal of excess cholesterol from the digestive tract. Inadequate fibre allows re-absorption into the circulatory system from the gut.

There are two types of fibre – soluble and insoluble. Soluble fibre is found in the soft pulp of fruits such as strawberries, peaches, nectarines and plums. Insoluble fibre is found in wholegrains and pulses (legumes) such as wild and brown rice, sweetcorn, black-eyed beans, kidney beans and lentils. Include at least two to three sources of either type of fibre every day.

### Good heart snacks

It is more beneficial for the heart for you to eat meals frequently rather than the traditional three meals a day. This is especially true of a heavy dinner, which exerts additional pressure on the heart to supply the rest of the body with the nutrients it needs. Good snacks include:

- Stewed apples and blackberries
- Grapefruit and orange-segment fruit salad
- Avocado dip on rye cakes
- Tahini (sesame seed dip) on oatcakes
- Sardines on Ryvita
- Salmon on buckwheat blinis
- Spinach salad with pine nuts
- Tuna and sweetcorn salad
- Lentil and carrot soup
- Mixed vegetable and barley soup

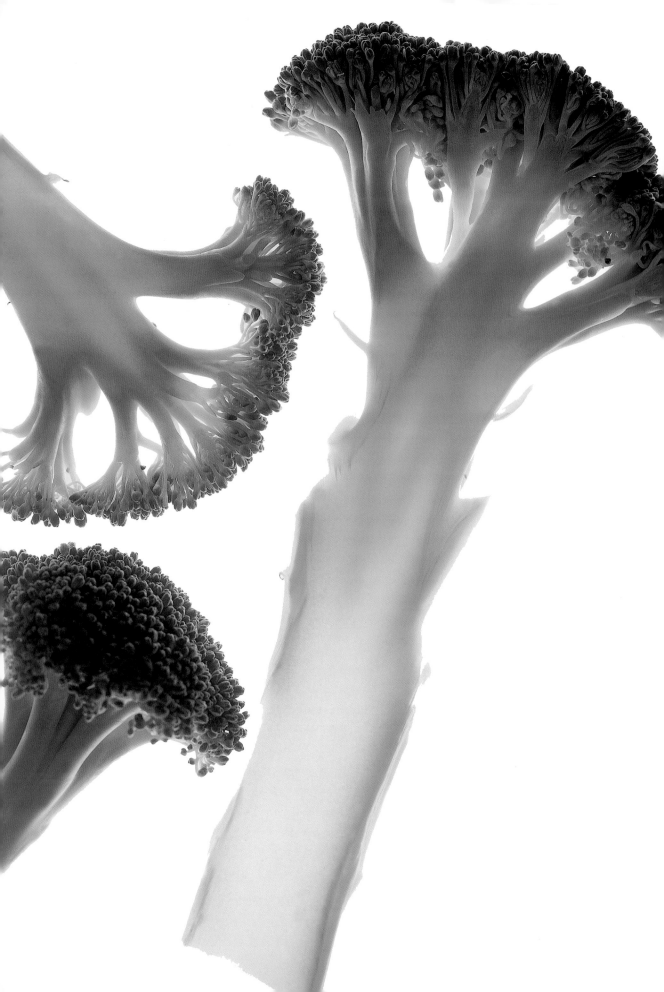

# cancer

Cancer is a blanket term for a group of over 100 different disease states. Some names are all too familiar, such as breast or lung cancer. These are very common diseases; other cancers, such as pancreatic cancer, are less well known because they have a lower incidence.

It is widely recognized that diet and lifestyle play an important role in the formation and spread of cancer. In this chapter we will examine how best to protect ourselves against cancer.

We all have cancerous cells within us, because they occur naturally. It is the job of the immune system (see pages 97–100) to clear them away. However, the creation of an environment conducive to the proliferation of these cells into what we know as cancer is largely up to us. We can influence our chances of getting the disease enormously through diet and lifestyle.

It is important to understand that nutrition consultants cannot, by law, 'treat' cancer. But we are often called in by a patient or their doctor to provide essential nutritional support. If a patient is being treated with conventional methods, then we can tailor a nutritional programme to reduce the side-effects. Some patients refuse chemotherapy, preferring more natural methods, in which case we can assist in creating a programme that will support their immune systems as fully as possible.

## How does cancer start?

Healthy cells replace themselves when they are damaged or worn out. This process of replication and replacement is usually carried out on a regular basis in a carefully controlled manner. Sometimes cells continue to replicate, but without control or order. The excess cells form new, independent tissue with its own blood supply, and this is the basis of a tumour. Many of these areas of new tissue are benign (posing no threat) and can be removed by surgery or left alone.

Some tumours are malignant. These are damaging because they contain cancerous cells that grow unchecked and can spread to other parts of the body to form more tumours.

Normal cells can become cancerous through exposure to carcinogens, or through genetic predisposition. The genes that are thought to have the ability to alter the characteristics of a cell are known as oncogenes. Oncogenes develop from normal genes called proto-oncogenes, which are involved in the day-to-day

LEFT Broccoli is part of the anti-cancer, cruciferous family of vegetables.

functioning of cells. Many factors can contribute to encouraging a proto-oncogene to become an oncogene, amongst them changes in DNA (see below), which is thought to mutate after contact with a carcinogen or virus. Oncogenes produce huge amounts of factors that stimulate the growth of mutated cells.

The growth of cancerous cells occurs for three main reasons: DNA damage, immune system problems and injury to cell membranes.

### DNA

Our genetic code is contained within a chemical called DNA. Each person's unique DNA make-up provides a blueprint for the manufacture of cells in the body. For example, if new cells are required in the digestive tract, the body knows what sort to create because it is programmed into the DNA.

However, if the DNA is damaged in any way, perhaps by free radicals, toxic chemicals or viruses, the formation of new cells can be adversely affected. To understand this, imagine a photocopier. If the original document fed into the machine has a blemish on it, the copies that are replicated will have the same blemish. If the machine is incorrectly programmed, it may produce 50 copies rather than the one copy you required. In a similar fashion, DNA sometimes produces too many damaged or immature cells. The extra cells then form a tumour.

### Immune system problems

The immune system is responsible for clearing away cell debris, in addition to cells that have not formed properly. You can read more about this in the section on the immune system (see pages 96–105). If the system is overworked, or not well supported by adequate nutrition, it becomes vulnerable. Mutant cells are not attacked and disposed of, allowing them to proliferate.

### Cell membranes

Through various mechanisms, the outer membrane layer of the cell can become damaged, leading to rapid cell division.

### Cancer triggers

Most of us have heard stories about people who have smoked 60 cigarettes a day for 70 years and never had a day of illness in their lives. It would seem that there are triggers that will set off the cancer process. These people obviously didn't have a trigger that responded to cigarette

| Common carcinogens | | |
| --- | --- | --- |
| • Smoking | • Burnt food | • Fried food |
| • Nitrates | • Nitrites | • Ultraviolet light |
| • Alcohol | • Radon gas | • Pesticides |
| • Asbestos | • Chlorine | • Fluoride |

smoke – nicotine and tobacco were not carcinogens for them. Perhaps their trigger was alcohol, and had they indulged in alcohol regularly, the outcome would have been different.

Some people may have more than one trigger, so cancer could result from any number of carcinogens, such as smoking, drinking alcohol and eating barbecued/burnt food, combined with a compromised immune system. Again, this underlines our biochemical individuality.

## Categories of cancer

There are many types of cancer, which fall into four main categories.

● **Leukaemias** are cancers of the tissue involved in the formation of blood, such as bone marrow. In this case, abnormal blood cells replicate out of control.

● **Carcinomas** are cancers that affect the layer of tissue that lines the external and internal surfaces of the body – the epithelium. The areas most at risk are glands, organs, skin and mucus membranes. The epithelial cells mutate, and are then produced too rapidly, and are often malformed in some way.

● **Sarcomas** are cancers that form in connective tissue and so can appear in any part of the body such as fat, muscle, blood or lymph.

● **Lymphomas** are cancers of the lymphatic system (see pages 121–122), which contains lymph – the fluid that 'bathes' body tissue. Lymph is filtered through the lymph nodes, whose role is to protect against infection and trap carcinogens, which makes them vulnerable to cancer.

| How does cancer grow? | |
|---|---|
| Initiation | The cells and tissue appear normal, yet minute changes are taking place within the cells. These changes initiate the process of cancer. |
| Promotion | The tissue alters as the new cells replicate out of control, forming a tumour. If, for any reason, the tissue were to be examined, the changes would be visible. |
| Progression | The cancer increases in size as more new cells are synthesized. The tumour now requires nutrients and oxygen of its own, so it creates a blood supply. This is done at the expense of the surrounding tissue. |
| Malignancy | The cancer has now taken hold and is unlikely to respond to any diet or lifestyle changes. Surgery, chemotherapy and radiology may be required to remove it. |
| Metastasis | The cancer migrates or travels to other parts of the body, leading to secondary tumours. |

### Free radicals, antioxidants and cancer

Free radicals are molecules that damage the body's DNA and cell membranes. They are closely linked to the initiation and spread of cancer. They are produced in the body as a normal by-product of metabolism. Sunlight, smoking and fried foods all create free radicals.

To disarm these potentially damaging free radicals, the body needs antioxidants. Imagine an apple cut into two halves, with lemon juice poured over one half and the other left as it is. After a few minutes, the untouched half will start to react with the oxygen in the air and turn

The body also manufactures its own antioxidants, such as two antioxidant enzymes produced in the liver, superoxide dismutase (SOD) and glutathione peroxidase (GP). These rely on nutrients for their formation. SOD is found in two forms: one requires manganese and iron, the other zinc and copper. GP requires selenium for its construction. All these minerals are found in fresh nuts and seeds, dark green leafy vegetables and wholegrain products. Including such foods in your meals every day should ensure that your body is supplied with the nutrients it needs to produce enough vital natural antioxidants.

'Prevention is better than cure', and we cannot ignore the importance of fresh food as part of a healthy lifestyle. Raw food can offer a greater level of all the nutrients, so get as much as you can, even if only in the form of fruit and juiced vegetables.

brown. The half covered in lemon juice will retain its original colour. The lemon juice has exerted a protective effect, acting as an antioxidant. The same sort of thing happens in the body, where antioxidants protect against damage by free radicals.

### Anti-cancer foods

The first step in protecting yourself against cancer is to reduce your exposure to things that promote free radicals: give up smoking, cover up in the sun and avoid fried foods. However, you can also help your body to maintain an adequate level of antioxidants, for example by eating foods containing antioxidant nutrients.

### Nutrition and cancer management

For those who already have cancer, good nutrition can play a powerful role in its management. There are three main nutritional aims: to support the immune system, to assist in detoxifying and protecting the body from the effects of the cancer and medical treatment, and to enhance the effects of conventional medicine, where possible.

Cancer cells thrive in oxygen-free environments. Good nutrition helps to defeat them by ensuring that all body tissues are well oxygenated. Cancer cells also flourish on arachadonic acid, which is one of the products of the metabolism of fats.

Some arachadonic acid is essential, but too much can encourage inflammation, in addition to creating a pro-cancerous environment. Excess arachadonic acid can often be avoided by removing saturated fats from the diet, such as full-fat milk, hard cheese and red meats. Eating lots of fresh fruit and vegetables, as well as fresh nuts, seeds and wholegrains, assists the successful conversion of fats into anti-inflammatory fats. Cancer cells are also thought to thrive in the sugar-rich environment created by a diet that is high in refined sugars and alcohol.

It is important to note one thing. We are not saying that a diet high in fats and sugars *will* lead to cancer, but that the risk will be increased if these foods are chosen instead of fresh foods that are thought to offer protection.

## Cancer treatment and nutrition

Treatments for cancer include surgery, hormone therapy, immunotherapy (boosting the body's own immune system with drugs), radiotherapy and chemotherapy. All these treatments tax the body, so having a first-class nutritional support regime is essential.

For example, during chemotherapy, chemicals are administered to attack the cancer cells. However, they also damage the surrounding healthy cells. Common side-effects range from hair loss and a drop in weight to confusion, depression and lethargy. Chemotherapy and radiotherapy are very demanding on the body and have a negative impact on the digestive system. Eating bland, well-cooked meals such as fish and vegetables, drinking aloe vera juice and supplementing with a probiotic helps to protect the digestive system through times of such treatments. We feel that it is imperative to support the immune system with optimum nutrition at this time.

It is important to understand some of the dietary principles that reduce the production of free radicals, and the environmental conditions that favour the development of cancers.

All body tissue has different levels of acidity and alkalinity but, overall, it functions best in a mildly alkaline state. Prolonged acidity within the body is pro-cancerous, and the typical Western diet (fried foods, food additives, colourings, sugar, salt, chemically treated food, excessive amounts of animal protein and dairy products) creates over-acidity.

High acidity can be combated by following a macrobiotic diet, which is highly alkaline. This means an abundant vegetable intake, low consumption of fats (avoiding all animal and dairy produce, which is high in saturated fats) and a regular intake of foods with properties known to reduce the development of cancers, such as soya beans, soya products and sea vegetables – seaweed, dulse and carrageen.

Cell function is regulated by a delicate balance of the minerals sodium and potassium. There is a greater amount of potassium inside each cell and a greater amount of sodium outside it. Together they create an electrical charge, not unlike that of a battery inside a torch. This is known as the sodium/potassium pump and it regulates which nutrients can enter the cell and which waste matter can leave it.

The Western diet is unhealthily high in salt, which is added to virtually every prepared foodstuff, primarily for 'taste' but also for its preservative action. This greatly disturbs the sodium/potassium pump, allowing for an increased possibility of cancer development. Max Gerson, who developed the Gerson method of naturopathic cancer treatment, advocated a high-potassium diet, similar to the diet our cavemen forefathers would have eaten. Potassium is found in abundance in raw, unprocessed plant foods, including all vegetables and fruits. Choose organic produce, which is free from chemicals, pesticides and fertilizers.

Balancing blood sugar levels is a vital part of cancer prevention. There is an increase in glucose metabolism with the onset of cancer, and this stimulates greater production of insulin. Once a cancer has started to develop, it will feed directly on blood glucose. Most importantly, the immune system is compromised by elevated levels of circulating blood glucose.

Saturated fats (found in animal produce) have a direct bearing on the development of cancer. Our cell membranes must remain fluid for the intake of nutrients and the clearing of toxic waste, in the same way as the sodium/potassium pump mentioned above. The most important nutrient for preventing the development of cancer is oxygen, as cancer cells cannot survive in the presence of it. But if you eat a lot of saturated fats, it causes the cell membranes to become rigid, inhibiting their uptake of oxygen. Abnormal cell development can then continue unchecked.

Fibre is essential for digestive health – and for the prevention of colon and rectal cancers. Many studies have looked at the influence of diet on different types of cancer, investigating both immediate and long-term effects.

Nitrites and nitrates are used to cure ham, beef, hot-dogs, bacon, sausages, fish and cooked meats. These contain similar carcinogenic compounds to those found in tobacco smoke. These types of food, in addition to barbecued and/or burnt foods, should be limited. The antioxidant vitamins A and E are especially important for neutralizing these damaging chemicals in the stomach, where nitrosamines are produced from nitrites and nitrates.

Alcohol has recently been found to be one of the most carcinogenic substances that we consume. Combined with smoking, its effects are increased many times over. While the occasional drink is acceptable, regular intake interferes with the process of detoxification by the liver and exposes the mouth, throat and oesophagus to potentially harmful chemicals. The picture is rather more serious for women than men because if liver detoxification is reduced or impeded excess oestrogens cannot be cleared efficiently and this may exacerbate the risk of the hormone-related cancers of the breast, ovaries and uterus.

## Environmental oestrogens

Many plastics and household products contain hormone-mimicking substances which have a similar biochemical structure to the oestrogen that our body produces. Synthetic oestrogens such as those found in the contraceptive pill and hormone replacement therapy (HRT) also have a much more powerful effect on oestrogen-sensitive tissue than the level of activity that natural oestrogen produces. These synthetic oestrogens have found their way into our water supply.

The hormone-mimicking substances and synthetic oestrogens, once in the body, fit into oestrogen-receptor sites and exert a powerful oestrogenic effect on body cells and tissues. This strong action initiates a rapid, out-of-control proliferation of cells which is thought to play a role in many oestrogen-receptive cancers such as breast, ovarian, endometrial and prostate cancer.

By avoiding the long-term use of synthetic oestrogens, using natural biodegradable cleaning products and avoiding wrapping or storing foods in plastic you can reduce your exposure to such oestrogens. Cruciferous vegetables and soya products also help to protect from oestrogen-receptive cancers.

## Anti-cancer foods

There are many foods that are now recognized to have potent anti-cancer properties. The saying that 'prevention is better than cure' could not be more applicable. With current estimations foretelling an incidence of the disease of almost one in two by 2005, we simply cannot ignore the importance of fresh food as part of a healthy lifestyle. Raw food will always offer a greater level of all the essential nutrients, so get as much as you can, if only in the form of fruit and juiced vegetables.

We are already familiar with the Fighting Five group of antioxidants which help the immune system function efficiently. These vitamins and minerals all play a vital role in preventing cancer cells from getting out of control. However, there are also other foods that have anti-cancer properties, and it is well worth including them in our daily diet.

## The cruciferous family

This group of foods includes broccoli, cauliflower, cabbage, Brussels sprouts, bok choy and watercress: all renowned as potent anti-cancer weapons. They contain indoles, which stimulate the production of the antioxidant enzyme glutathione peroxidase. It is believed that indoles inactivate excess oestrogens, which can cause cancer, particularly of the breast. These vegetables also contain good levels of vitamin C, a potent antioxidant, and should be eaten raw wherever possible to preserve their indole content, or lightly steamed.

## Soya beans and soya products

Soya beans and any products made from them, such as tofu, tempeh, miso and soy sauce, prevent abnormal cell growth. They also contain isoflavones and phyto-oestrogens, both of which have anti-cancer properties. A further benefit is that these foods have been found to reduce the toxic side-effects of chemotherapy and radiation.

### Garlic and onions

Garlic acts as a chelator, which means that it latches on to and carries away toxins from the body, including potentially cancerous heavy metals such as cadmium from cigarettes. Onions behave in the same way as garlic, although to a lesser degree. They both contain allicin, a sulphur compound which is a potent detoxifier. In addition, garlic stimulates the white blood cells that consume cancer cells.

One of the commonest forms of cancer is stomach cancer, but a regular intake of both garlic and onions can reduce the likelihood of developing this disease. Garlic is also a rich source of sulphur, required by the liver for effective detoxification. As the liver is the clearing-house for all potentially cancer-forming chemicals and pathogens passing through the body, the importance of this humble vegetable cannot be underestimated.

### Kelp

Kelp contains a rich source of iodine, which is essential for the health of the thyroid, the gland that regulates blood sugar (energy) metabolism. It is well-known that the thyroid starts to shrink from the mid-twenties onwards and many people are found to have hypothyroidism (insufficient production of thyroid hormones) from this time.

If energy production is lowered, the body's blood sugar metabolism alters to adapt, which can be pro-cancerous. Kelp contains abundant amounts of selenium, which is a potent antioxidant. (See Heart Nutrition, page 132.)

### Almonds

These nuts contain leatrile, a natural compound that contains a cyanide-like substance deadly to cancer cells. The ancient Greeks, Romans, Egyptians and Chinese all consumed seeds and stones from fruits such as apricots, as they believed them to have anti-cancer properties. Conventionally, leatrile has been used as an anti-cancer treatment, but not as a food source.

### Oriental mushrooms

Maitake, shiitake and rei-shi mushrooms contain powerful, immune-stimulating polysaccharides known as beta-glucans. These are not found in ordinary mushrooms, so it is worth seeking out these Eastern gems, even in dried form, from supermarkets and Chinese food shops. Use them in any recipe that calls for mushrooms.

### Tomatoes

These fruits have received much recognition in the last few years for their anti-cancer properties. They are rich in lycopene, a powerful antioxidant which is believed to be more effective than vitamin A and beta-carotene.

## Carrots

Like most orange-coloured vegetables, carrots are one of the richest sources of beta-carotene, the precursor to vitamin A, one of the Fighting Five antioxidants. The craze for consuming large amounts of juiced carrots as a cancer therapy, especially to treat breast cancer, misses an important point: a large amount of essential nutrients are lost in the juicing process, not to mention fibre. It is necessary to eat plenty of raw carrots as well as juicing them.

## Citrus fruits

Citrus fruits and cranberries contain bioflavonoids: these support and boost the antioxidant quality of vitamin C, which these fruits have in rich supply.

## Peppers

These contain capsaicin, which is believed to block the cancer-forming compounds found in smoked and cured meats and fish. Peppers are also an excellent source of beta-carotene, particularly red peppers.

## Seeds

Linseeds, pumpkin seeds, sunflower seeds and sesame seeds all contain lignans, compounds that are found in the tough outer husk of the seed. Lignans are phyto-oestrogens (that is, they block the action of harmful environmental and synthetic oestrogens) and may help reduce excess oestrogens circulating in the body – the excess oestrogens are known to stimulate hormone-based cancers, such as breast cancer, ovarian cancer and uterine cancer.

Eating one tablespoon per day of these mixed seeds is thought to be beneficial. Mix the seeds with 'smoothies' (see the recipes on pages 146–171), and try them in fruit salads, and in fruit juices on cereals (granolas). You can also add them to salads, soups and stews. Soya beans, tofu, miso and tempeh are all good sources of lignans, which could be one of the reasons why the Asian countries have a lower incidence of hormone-related cancers.

## Raw power

The benefits of raw food in cancer prevention is vital. Ideally, at least 50 per cent of daily intake should be raw. Juiced fruit and vegetables are excellent, as they contain a condensed level of all the antioxidant nutrients, but these should be complemented by raw salads, vegetable crudités and fruits to help eliminate toxins from the digestive tract.

### Beta-carotene foods

The carotenoid family of fruits and vegetables are rich in beta-carotene, an essential part of the antioxidant team.

The richest sources of these are oranges, lemons, cantaloupe melons, mangoes, papayas, tomatoes, red, yellow and green peppers, carrots, kale, broccoli, spring greens, spinach, collards, squash, sweet potatoes, apricots and peaches.

# Recipes

## Recipes for a healthy digestive system

Raw and fresh fruit and vegetables all contain digestive enzymes, which reduce the digestive load on the body. Raw juices are particularly beneficial. Onions, garlic and rice are all known to have a calming effect on the digestive system as a whole and, even in the most severe cases of digestive disruption, any of these three foods can have a settling effect. The fibre found in fruit, vegetables and wholegrains is important for maintaining proper bowel function, and preventing constipation.

### SCRAMBLED EGGS ON A BED OF SPINACH

If you suffer from digestive problems such as indigestion, bloating and wind then you may find that some protein-rich meals are difficult to digest. Eggs, however, are a great source of quality protein, and scrambling them helps to break down the protein, making them much easier to digest. Spinach is rich in calcium and magnesium, which are needed by the muscles that move food through the intestine, making this a perfect digestive start to the day.

**Ingredients**

4 organic or free-range eggs
125ml (4floz) milk or soya milk
Black pepper

450g (1lb) fresh or frozen spinach
1 teaspoon olive oil
1 tablespoon finely chopped fresh parsley

**Method**

Crack the eggs into a bowl and whisk with a fork until a smooth consistency is reached. Whisk in the milk and black pepper. Wash and drain the spinach, then steam or cook it in just the water that clings to the leaves after washing. Drain the spinach. Heat the oil in a non-stick frying pan and pour in the egg mixture. Stir continuously until the mixture sets and thickens, then take the pan off the heat and leave to stand while you divide the spinach between four plates. Spoon the scrambled eggs on top of the bed of spinach and sprinkle with parsley.

### PINEAPPLE AND PAPAYA SMOOTHIE

These two tropical fruits are laden with enzymes that can aid digestion and reduce inflammation. Natural bio yoghurt is packed full of friendly bacteria that help to keep your small intestine and colon healthy. Excellent as a quick and easy breakfast.

**Ingredients**

½ of a fresh pineapple
1 ripe papaya
4 ice cubes
250ml (8floz) rice or soya milk

2 tablespoons cow's milk or
  bio soya yoghurt
1 tablespoon coconut milk

**Method**

Peel and chop the pineapple and place in a blender. Peel and de-seed the papaya and add to the blender. Add the ice cubes, rice or soya milk, cow's milk or bio soya yoghurt and the coconut milk and blend on a high speed until smooth. Serve chilled.

Breakfasts

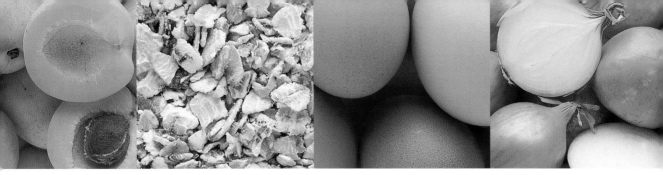

## HIGH-FIBRE PORRIDGE

Oats help to stabilize blood sugar levels by providing a sustained source of energy. Oats and oat bran are rich in soluble fibre which increases intestinal muscle tone and acts as a good food source for all those friendly gut bacteria. This high-fibre start to the day can really help to keep you more regular.

**Ingredients**

4 prunes (stoned)

8 tablespoons porridge oats

600ml (1 pint) water

2 tablespoons oat bran

2 teaspoons black strap molasses (optional)

**Method**

Place all the ingredients in a saucepan and bring to the boil slowly on a moderate heat, stirring frequently. You will find that the mixture starts to thicken as it comes to the boil. Simmer for 2–3 minutes then dilute to the desired consistency with milk or water if it is too thick. Serve hot.

## CABBAGE AND APPLE TONIC

The benefits of fresh raw fruit and vegetable juicing on digestion are numerous. If you are lucky enough to own a juice extractor, it is time to put it to good use. This may sound like an unappealing combination, but it is in fact very pleasant. Cabbage juice has remarkable healing properties for the intestinal lining, while apple is good for reactivating beneficial gut bacteria and relieving constipation. This is an excellent digestive tonic and is suitable for sufferers of diarrhoea, colitis, coeliac and Crohn's disease.

**Ingredients**

4 cooking apples

¼ of a white cabbage

8 ice cubes

4 sprigs of mint

**Method**

Wash and core the apples. Peel off and discard the outer layers of the white cabbage. Push the cabbage and apple through a juicer. Pour into four glasses, add the ice cubes and serve with a sprig of mint.

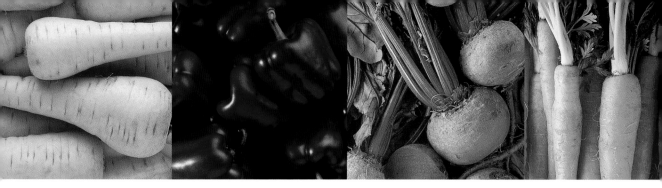

## FENNEL AND CELERY SOUP

Both these vegetables are good digestive healers. Celery helps to support liver function whilst fennel soothes an inflamed digestive lining. When experiencing digestive problems it is important not to eat too much raw food, so well-cooked vegetables in the form of nourishing soups and stews are great as they give the digestive system time to heal and recover.

**Ingredients**

| | |
|---|---|
| 1 large brown onion | 600ml (1 pint) vegetable stock |
| 450g (1lb) potatoes | 1 tablespoon fresh thyme |
| 2 bulbs of root fennel | 2 bay leaves |
| 1 head of celery | 1 tablespoon finely chopped fresh parsley |

**Method** Peel and chop the onion and potatoes. Wash and finely chop the fennel and celery. Place all the ingredients in a large heavy-based saucepan, bring to the boil and boil for 10 minutes. Cover the pan, reduce the heat and simmer for a further 30 minutes. Remove from the heat and allow to cool slightly. Remove and discard the bay leaves then put the contents into a blender or food processor. Blend until smooth, pour back into the saucepan and reheat. Pour into soup bowls and sprinkle with parsley. Delicious with toasted rye bread.

## SWEET POTATO SURPRISE

Sweet potatoes are easy to digest and rich in beta-carotene hence their distinctive colour. Beta-carotene is converted into vitamin A, a powerful antioxidant that helps to reduce intestinal inflammation. Goat's cheese is a great alternative to cheese made from cow's milk, which you may be avoiding if following a dairy-free diet. The sweet taste of the potatoes complements the strong flavour of the goat's cheese, and this dish acts as a highly nutritious replacement for the standard lunch of baked potato and cheddar cheese.

**Ingredients**

| | |
|---|---|
| 4 large sweet potatoes | 1 tablespoon pine nuts |
| 300g (10½oz) soft goat's cheese | |

**Method** Preheat the oven to 220°C/425°F/Gas 7. Wash the sweet potatoes, place on a baking tray and put in the centre of the oven. Bake for 30–40 minutes or until cooked (when cooked a sharp knife will slide easily into the centre of the potato). Remove from the oven, slit lengthways and carefully remove the cooked flesh from the skin, reserving the skins. Mix the sweet potato flesh with the goat's cheese and pine nuts then pack it back into the skins. Return to the oven for a further 5 minutes or until the goat's cheese has melted. Serve with a green leafy salad for a perfect light lunch.

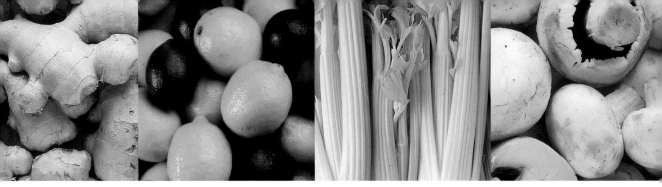

## MINTY YOGHURT DRESSING OR DIP

Bloating and pain after eating is often caused when intestinal muscle spasms create trapped wind, and mint is reputed to have benefits for a painful, swollen stomach. The essential oils in peppermint can also help relax intestinal muscles thus reducing bloating. This is deliciously refreshing as a dip with crudités or can be thinned down with olive oil and lemon juice for a salad dressing.

**Ingredients**

1 tablespoon fresh mint
1 spring onion
125ml (4floz) natural bio yoghurt

For a salad dressing:
1 tablespoon olive oil
Juice of ½ lemon

**Method**

Wash and finely chop the mint and spring onion. In a bowl, mix together the yoghurt, mint and spring onion and stir thoroughly. If you want, you can now use this as a dip – simply garnish with a couple of fresh mint leaves. If you want to use this as a dressing add the olive oil and lemon juice and mix well then serve with a green salad.

## OVEN-STEAMED SNAPPER

The average adult digestive lining is over 9 metres (30 feet) long, and requires both protein and zinc for its maintenance and repair. White fish is easy to digest and provides an excellent source of both these nutrients. This dish is simple, quick to prepare and delicious.

**Ingredients**

2 whole red snapper
  or sea bass (gutted)
1 tablespoon chopped fresh parsley
1 tablespoon fresh marjoram
1 tablespoon fresh thyme
4 large potatoes
6 shallots

1 tablespoon olive oil
2 cloves of garlic
10 cherry tomatoes
Black pepper
300ml (½ pint) vegetable stock
1 teaspoon anchovy essence
Juice of ½ lemon

**Method**

Preheat the oven to 200°C/400°F/Gas 6. Wash the fish and stuff with half of the parsley, marjoram and thyme. Wash, peel, thinly slice and parboil the potatoes for 10 minutes, then drain and leave to cool. Peel and finely chop the shallots and garlic. Use half the olive oil to grease a deep baking tray. Lay the sliced potatoes, shallots and garlic on the bottom. Lay the fish on top. Scatter on the tomatoes, the rest of the herbs and olive oil and a pinch of black pepper. Mix together the vegetable stock, anchovy essence and lemon juice and pour over the fish. Cover with foil and bake for 30–40 minutes. Serve with a slice of lemon.

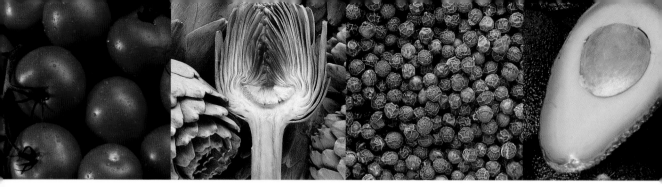

## MOROCCAN LAMB WITH CORIANDER QUINOA

This aromatic dish is full of digestive tonics. Turmeric and ginger possess powerful anti-inflammatory properties whilst apricots are rich in beta-carotene, important for the health of the mucus membranes that line the digestive tract. Fresh parsley is rich in vitamin C and iron, and coriander binds with toxins encouraging efficient cleansing. Moroccan lamb dishes are usually served with couscous, a wheat product that can contribute to digestive problems, so we suggest using quinoa instead, a South American grain that makes an excellent alternative to couscous and is usually very well tolerated by those with sensitive digestion.

**Ingredients**

1 large brown onion
300g (10½oz) potatoes
1 tablespoon olive oil
450g (1lb) lean diced lamb
1 teaspoon ground coriander
½ teaspoon ground cumin
1 teaspoon grated fresh ginger
2 cloves of garlic
250ml (8floz) vegetable stock

240g (8½oz) chickpeas
8 fresh or dried apricots
Black pepper
1 tablespoon chopped fresh parsley
400g (14oz) quinoa
½ teaspoon ground turmeric
6 large tomatoes chopped
1 tablespoon chopped fresh coriander

**Method**

Preheat the oven to 180°C/350°F/Gas 4. Peel and chop the onion, garlic and potatoes. In a large ovenproof casserole dish, heat the olive oil until just smoking. Add the lamb and onion and cook on a high heat to sear the lamb and sweat the onions. When the lamb is brown, reduce the heat and stir in the coriander, cumin, ginger and garlic and cook for a couple of minutes. Add the stock, chickpeas, potatoes, apricots and a pinch of pepper. Cover the dish and place in the oven for 1 hour or until the lamb is tender. Check after 40 minutes and top up with a little water if the stew is looking too dry. Remove from the oven, stir in the parsley, then replace the lid and allow the meat to rest for 10 minutes. Meanwhile, rinse the quinoa then add it and the turmeric to a saucepan full of boiling water. Cook for 10–15 minutes or until the quinoa is swollen and soft. Drain the quinoa, stir in the tomatoes and coriander and season with black pepper. Serve the quinoa and Moroccan lamb hot.

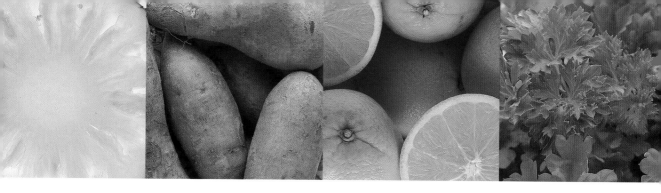

## SPICY APPLE AND PEAR FOOL

Naturally sweet and high in the soluble fibre pectin, this dish makes a healthy dessert for anyone. Pectin helps to improve bowel regularity and binds with toxins and heavy metals ensuring safe elimination from the body.

**Ingredients**
4 cooking apples
4 ripe pears
100ml (3½floz) water

1 teaspoon honey
½ teaspoon cinnamon
200ml (7floz) soya cream

**Method**
Peel, core and chop the apples and pears and add to a saucepan with the water, honey and cinnamon. Bring to the boil then reduce the heat and simmer until the fruit is soft and fluffy, which should take about 5 –10 minutes. Remove from the heat and leave to cool. Stir in the soya cream, pour into individual pudding pots and place in the fridge to chill.

## DAIRY-FREE RICE PUDDING

Everyone loves this old-fashioned pudding, which is a great accompaniment to any fresh stewed fruit. Making a dairy-free version is simple – all you do is swap the traditional cow's milk for unsweetened soya or rice milk. This is a dish that you can be creative with – experiment by adding different ingredients such as prunes, apricots, blueberries, raspberries, cocoa powder or sesame seeds.

**Ingredients**
225g (8oz) brown rice
600ml (1 pint) rice or soya milk
½ teaspoon vanilla extract

1 organic or free-range egg
Nutmeg

**Method**
Preheat the oven to 180°C/350°F/Gas 4. Grease an ovenproof casserole dish. Rinse the rice. In a saucepan, bring the milk to the boil and add the rice and vanilla extract. Turn down the heat, cover the pan and simmer for 40–50 minutes or until the rice is soft. Check frequently and add more milk if it becomes too dry. Stir occasionally to prevent the rice from sticking to the bottom of the pan. When the rice is cooked beat the egg with a fork in a bowl. Remove the pan from the heat and stir in the beaten egg then pour the mixture into the casserole dish. Grate nutmeg over the top of the pudding and place in the oven for 20–30 minutes, until golden brown. Serve piping hot.

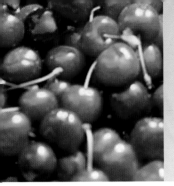
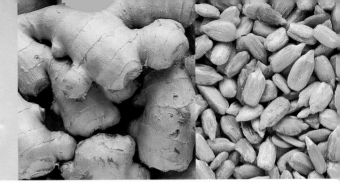

# Recipes to help the immune system

Stimulants such as tea, coffee and alcohol, recreational and prescription drugs, and pollution all induce the production of free radicals. A strong immune system will combat disease on a daily basis, providing it is well supported. Foods rich in antioxidant nutrients – vitamins A, C, E, and the minerals zinc and selenium – are found in fresh fruits, vegetables, fish, wholegrains, nuts and seeds.

### AVOCADO AND KIWI FRUIT SMOOTHIE

This wake-up drink is packed full of immune-boosting nutrients. Avocados are rich in vitamin E, which protects cells against the harmful effects of toxins and helps vitamin C work more efficiently. Kiwi fruit and lime juice are rich in vitamin C, the top nutrient for immune protection; and coconut milk is rich in lauric acid, believed to have antiviral properties. All in all, a great way to start the day.

**Ingredients**

4 kiwi fruit
1 avocado
Juice of ½ lime

300ml (½ pint) rice or soya milk
60ml (2floz) coconut milk, plus extra to swirl
4 ice cubes

**Method**

Peel the kiwi fruit and place in a blender. Peel and de-stone the avocado and add to the blender with all the other ingredients. Blend on a high speed until smooth. Pour into glasses and serve with a swirl of coconut milk on top.

### CHERRY BREAKFAST

Black cherries taste delicious and are high in bioflavanols and vitamin C, both potent antioxidants. Cherries are good for cleansing the blood and aiding elimination, making this a great start to a morning after a night before. Sunflower seeds add in essential fatty acids, which are also important for immune function. The oats contain fibre and are a good source of slow-release carbohydrate, which provides you with the energy you need to make it through a busy morning.

**Ingredients**

400g (14oz) stoned black cherries
    (fresh, frozen or tinned)
200g (7oz) tofu or 175ml (6floz)
    natural bio yoghurt

2 tablespoons sunflower seeds
1 litre (1¾ pints) rice or soya milk
3 tablespoons porridge oats

**Method**

Place all the ingredients in a blender and blend on a high speed until smooth. Serve straight away.

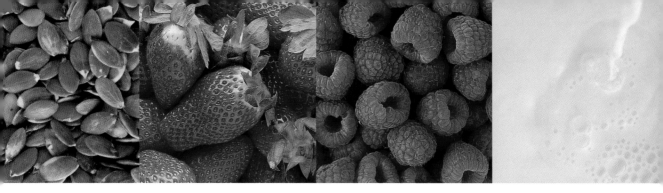

## BEETROOT SOUP

Bioflavanols and pro-anthocyanadins are found in purple fruits and vegetables. These little plant nutrients are powerful immune-boosters and have antiviral properties. They are also important for the integrity of veins, arteries and capillaries through which many of the immune cells travel. Beetroot has similar properties, making this soup a great tonic if you have an infection or are simply feeling a little under the weather.

**Ingredients**

450g (1lb) potatoes
3 beetroot
1 large brown onion
2 cloves of garlic
600ml (1 pint) vegetable stock

Sprig of fresh rosemary
2 teaspoons balsamic vinegar
60ml (2floz) natural bio yoghurt
Black pepper

**Method**

Peel and chop the potatoes, beetroot, onion and garlic. Add to a large saucepan with the stock, rosemary and balsamic vinegar and bring to the boil. Reduce the heat and simmer for 45 minutes. Remove from the heat and allow to cool slightly then remove and discard the rosemary sprig. Pour the contents into a blender or food processor and blend until smooth. Add the yoghurt and season to taste with pepper. Reheat gently then serve.

## PARSLEY AND LEEK SOUP

Parsley is very high in vitamin C and magnesium. Vitamin C provides cellular protection from free-radical damage and magnesium is important for the spleen, a body organ that is involved with immune cell production and storage. Leeks also have a reputation for being good cleansers whilst encouraging the elimination of uric acid, an acid that is closely linked to gout and muscle pains.

**Ingredients**

1 large bunch of parsley
450g (1lb) potatoes
4 leeks

1 brown onion
240g (8½oz) butter beans
600ml (1 pint) vegetable stock

**Method**

Wash and chop the parsley. Wash, peel and chop the potatoes and leeks. Peel and chop the onion. Place all the ingredients in a large saucepan and bring to the boil. Turn down the heat and simmer for 40 minutes. Serve in soup bowls with a sprinkling of fresh chopped parsley.

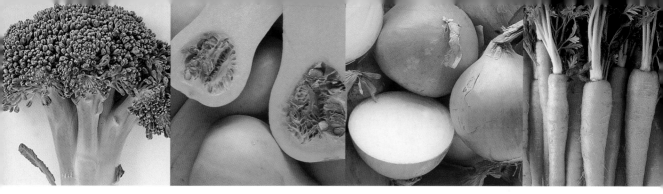

## WARM TURKEY AND WATERCRESS SALAD

This is a fantastic immune-boosting salad. Watercress is one of the top ten best antioxidant foods, being rich in vitamin C, magnesium and beta-carotene, and is an essential food for cellular protection, detoxification and anti-microbial activity. Added to which, being rich in potassium, watercress improves kidney function and helps to clear excess phlegm and mucus.

**Ingredients**

| | |
|---|---|
| Handful of baby spinach | 4 red onions |
| Handful of radicchio | 1 tablespoon olive oil |
| Handful of little gem leaves | 450g (1lb) turkey breast |
| 1 bunch of watercress | 1 clove of garlic |
| 1 courgette | 1 tablespoon sesame seeds |
| ½ cucumber | cranberry dressing (see recipe below) |

**Method**

Preheat the grill. Wash all the salad leaves, dry well and tear up into small pieces. Wash the watercress and add to the salad leaves. Wash and slice into strips the courgette and cucumber. Mix the salad leaves, courgette and cucumber and place a large handful on each plate. Peel and slice the red onions into rings, place on a shallow baking tray and drizzle with olive oil. Slice up the turkey meat and peel and chop the garlic, then lay these over the onion. Place under a hot grill for 10 minutes then turn the turkey over and cook for a further 5–10 minutes or until the turkey is cooked through. Spoon the turkey and onions onto the salad leaves, sprinkle with sesame seeds and drizzle with cranberry dressing.

## CRANBERRY DRESSING

Cranberries are loaded with bioflavanols, plant chemicals that act as powerful immune stimulators. Cranberries have long been known to have anti-bacterial properties and are particularly effective at protecting the bladder and kidneys from bacterial infection.

**Ingredients**

| | |
|---|---|
| 1 tablespoon cranberry sauce or jelly (preferably unsweetened) | 5 tablespoons olive oil |
| 2 tablespoons red wine vinegar | Pinch of black pepper |

**Method**

Place all the ingredients in a screw-top jar and shake well. Chill and use as a salad dressing. The dressing should keep for up to 1 month if refrigerated.

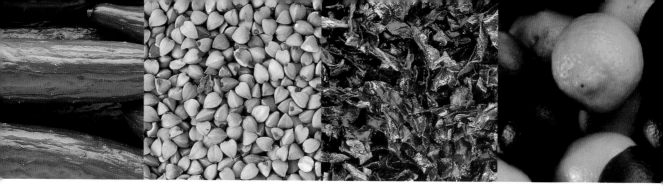

## PUMPKIN SEED BUTTER

This is pure indulgence. A very rich seed butter that can be used to spread on rice cakes, oatcakes or rye crackers for a quick snack that is rich in protein and zinc. Both these nutrients are vital for immune function whilst pumpkin seeds are one of the richest sources of zinc and have long been associated with immune protection, prostate protection and fertility. Pumpkin seeds are also rich in the essential omega-6 oils that are vital for immune and lymphatic function.

**Ingredients**
200g (7oz) pumpkin seeds
150–200ml (5–7floz) olive oil

**Method**
Grind the pumpkin seeds to a powder consistency. This is easiest in the coffee grinder attachment of a food processor. Transfer to a bowl and add the olive oil, 1 teaspoon at a time, until you get a good spreading consistency, like that of peanut butter. Keep in the refrigerator in a screw-top jar for freshness – it will keep for up to 1 week.

## WALNUT, AUBERGINE AND TOFU PÂTÉ

Walnuts are rich in the antioxidants vitamins C and E, a combination that works to protect our cells from the damaging and ageing effects of toxins and pollutants. Walnuts are also rich in the immune-boosting mineral zinc, required for the manufacture of T-cells by the thymus gland.

**Ingredients**
1 aubergine
1 small red onion
1 clove of garlic
1 tablespoon olive oil
2 teaspoons mixed dried herbs

1 tablespoon tomato purée
200g (7oz) walnuts
250g (9oz) plain tofu
Juice of 1 lemon
Black pepper

**Method**
Chop the aubergine into small cubes. Peel and finely chop the onion and garlic. Heat the olive oil in a frying pan and gently fry the onion until soft and translucent. Turn down the heat and add the garlic, aubergine, herbs and tomato purée and fry until the aubergine is cooked. Add a little water if it becomes too dry, then leave to cool slightly. Crush the walnuts to a powder in a blender or food processor and set to one side. Place all the fried ingredients and the tofu into the blender or food processor and blend on a high speed until smooth. Add water if needed. Slowly add the powdered walnuts, adding more water if needed to make a fairly thick consistency. Season to taste with lemon juice and pepper. This pâté can be used at lunchtime to accompany salads, fill baked potatoes or simply as a snack on rice cakes, oatcakes or rye crackers.

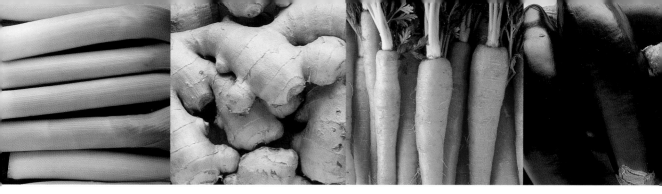

## MEDITERRANEAN SARDINES

The lymphatic system requires a good supply of omega-3 essential fatty acids for optimum function and immunity. Sardines are part of the oily fish family, which means they are rich in these immune-protecting omega-3 oils. Garlic helps to fight infections whilst tomatoes and peppers contain antioxidants that help to boost cellular protection.

**Ingredients**

8 fresh sardines (gutted)
2 red peppers
1 yellow pepper
2 medium red chillies
2 courgettes
1 aubergine
6 shallots
2 cloves of garlic

15 cherry tomatoes
1 tablespoon chopped fresh basil
1 tablespoon chopped fresh thyme
1 tablespoon chopped fresh marjoram
1 tablespoon chopped fresh oregano
2 tablespoons olive oil
Black pepper

**Method**

Preheat the oven to 200°C/400°F/Gas 6. Wash the sardines and remove the heads and tails. Wash, slice and de-seed the peppers and chillies. Wash and slice the courgettes and aubergine and place on a deep greased baking tray. Peel and chop the shallots and garlic and add to the baking tray. Add the cherry tomatoes. Sprinkle the herbs over the vegetables and drizzle with the olive oil. Lay the fish on top, sprinkle with black pepper and bake in the oven for 20 minutes. Serve with a green salad.

## SUN-DRIED TOMATO TUNA

Tuna is another member of the oily fish family, and for this recipe you need fresh tuna steaks not tinned tuna. Tomatoes are rich in beta-carotene and lycopene, another antioxidant from the carotene group, which helps to protect eye tissue.

**Ingredients**

1 red onion
2 cloves of garlic
1 red pepper
1 orange pepper

2 tablespoons olive oil
4 medium tuna steaks
4 heaped teaspoons sun-dried tomato pesto

**Method**

Preheat the oven to 200°C/400°F/Gas 6. Peel and chop the onion and garlic. Wash, de-seed and slice the peppers. Heat the olive oil in a large heavy-based frying pan, add the onion, garlic and peppers and quickly fry until lightly browned. Transfer to an ovenproof dish and place the tuna on top. Put a heaped teaspoon of sun-dried tomato pesto on top of each tuna steak. Cover the dish and bake in the oven for 15–20 minutes. Serve with a fresh green salad and new potatoes.

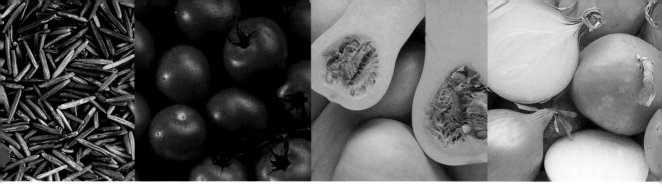

## THAI-STYLE PRAWNS

Unfortunately, years of intensive agriculture has left our soil depleted of many minerals. One mineral that has suffered a major drop is selenium, which is especially important for the function of the immune system. Some researchers attribute the rise in many cancers with the decline in selenium in our diets. Luckily prawns remain high in selenium and zinc, the two immune-strengthening minerals. Prawns are easy to digest and high in protein, which is essential for healing and repairing damaged body tissue. This is a really simple and quick meal.

**Ingredients**

6 spring onions
1 clove of garlic
1 red chilli
1 tablespoon olive oil
½ teaspoon Thai red curry paste

1 teaspoon grated fresh ginger
700g (1½ lb) large fresh or frozen prawns
125ml (4floz) coconut milk
½ teaspoon oyster sauce
1 tablespoon chopped fresh coriander

**Method**

Peel and chop the spring onions and garlic. Chop and de-seed the chilli. Heat the oil in a large frying pan and add the red curry paste, onions, garlic, chilli and ginger and cook for 1–2 minutes. Add the prawns and cook for a further 4 minutes, turning the prawns all the time. Add the coconut milk, oyster sauce and coriander and cook for a further 3–5 minutes. Serve on a bed of rice or buckwheat noodles.

## SUMMER SIX DELIGHT

Purple and red berries are packed full of nature's immune boosters – bioflavanols, pro-anthocyanadins and vitamin C. These plant chemicals give them their characteristic red, purple and blue colours. Luckily, you don't have to wait until summer for this delicious dessert. You can use frozen or tinned berries (in natural juice not sweetened syrup) all year round.

**Ingredients**

100g (3½oz) blackcurrants
100g (3½oz) raspberries
100g (3½oz) black cherries
100g (3½oz) strawberries
100g (3½oz) blackberries

100g (3½oz) blueberries
2 teaspoons honey
175ml (6floz) water
4 star anise

**Method**

Rinse all the fruit and place in a heavy-based saucepan with all the other ingredients. Bring to the boil, stirring continuously, then turn down the heat and simmer for 1–2 minutes. Leave to cool slightly then remove the star anise. Serve hot or cold with home-made rice pudding (see page 151) or natural yoghurt.

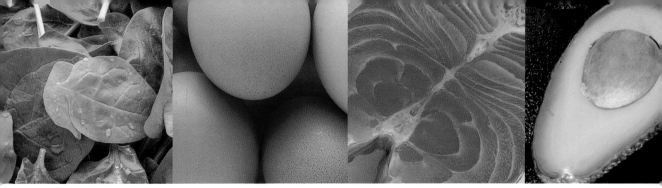

# Recipes to reduce inflammation

The omega-3 group of essential fatty acids found in nuts, seeds and oily fish all contain potent anti-inflammatory compounds. Various fruits and vegetables from the nightshade family, however, including tomatoes, potatoes, aubergines and courgettes (zucchini), have the opposite effect, contributing to the pain and inflammation associated with such conditions as rheumatoid arthritis. Free radicals are an inevitable by-product of inflammation and may be reduced by including plenty of antioxidant-rich foods such as those found in red, yellow and orange fruits and vegetables, nuts, seeds and wholegrains.

### PINK PANTHER

This is a very refreshing wake-up drink. Lime juice is high in vitamin C, which has natural anti-histamine properties, helping to combat inflammation. When the body is in a state of inflammation it is often too acidic and cranberries are highly alkaline, helping to restore the body's natural balance. The pink flesh and black seeds of the watermelon are rich in antioxidants, which help to protect cells from the damaging effects of cellular inflammation.

**Ingredients**
1 litre (1¾ pints) apple
   and cranberry juice
6 ice cubes

½ of a watermelon
2 bananas
Juice of 1 lime

**Method**
Place all the ingredients (including the seeds of the watermelon) in a blender and blend on a high speed until smooth. Pour into glasses and serve straight away.

### MACKEREL PÂTÉ

Mackerel is one of the richest sources of omega-3 essential fatty acids. These fatty acids are converted into hormone-like substances capable of counterbalancing pain and inflammation. This pâté can be used either at lunchtime on rye toast with salad, or as an excellent snack on oatcakes, rice cakes or rye crackers.

**Ingredients**
2 fresh mackerel fillets, cooked
   and de-boned
1 tablespoon creamed horseradish

1 tablespoon natural bio yoghurt
Juice of 1 lemon
Black pepper

**Method**
Remove the silvery grey skin from the mackerel and discard. Use a fork to break up the fish in a bowl. Add the horseradish, yoghurt and lemon juice. Continue to mix until smooth. If the pâté is too stiff add more yoghurt. Season to taste with black pepper.

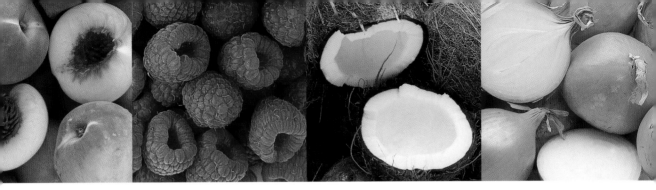

## CARROT AND SWEET POTATO SOUP

Carrots are rich in beta-carotene, which the body converts into the immune-boosting antioxidant vitamin A. Carrots support liver and kidney function making them excellent for detoxification. These brightly coloured vegetables also have antiviral and antibacterial properties boosting your protection against infection. Coriander is a good blood cleanser and ginger is known to be anti-inflammatory. Orange juice is rich in vitamin C, a vital nutrient for cellular protection.

**Ingredients**
450g (1lb) carrots
450g (1lb) sweet potatoes
3 sticks of celery
1 large brown onion

2.5cm (1in) fresh ginger
1 tablespoon chopped fresh coriander
600ml (1 pint) vegetable stock
Juice of 1 orange

**Method**
Wash, peel and chop the carrots and sweet potatoes. Wash and chop the celery. Peel and chop the onion. Grate the ginger. Place all the ingredients in a large saucepan and bring to the boil, then turn down the heat and simmer for 30 minutes. Remove from the heat and allow to cool slightly then pour the contents into a blender or food processor and blend until smooth. Return to the saucepan to reheat, then pour into bowls and serve with a sprinkling of coriander.

## FLAX OIL DRESSING

Flax is one of the most important anti-inflammatory foods. It is particularly useful for vegetarians and vegans as it is the richest appropriate source of omega-3 essential fatty acids. Keeping a jar of this dressing in your fridge to use over salads is the best way to keep your omega-3 levels topped up if you don't eat oily fish. Flax oil is available from most good health food shops.

**Ingredients**
1 clove of garlic
5 tablespoons flax oil
2 tablespoons white wine
  vinegar, balsamic vinegar
  or lemon juice

1 teaspoon honey
1 teaspoon wholegrain Dijon mustard
Pinch of black pepper

**Method**
Peel the garlic and slice in half. Place all the ingredients in a screw-top jar and shake well until all the ingredients have blended. Use drizzled over salads.

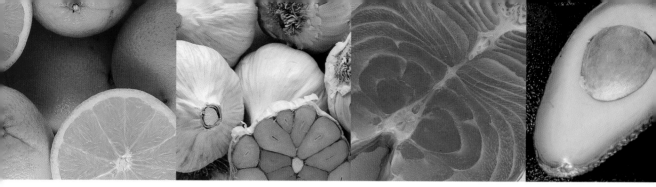

## STEAMED VEGETABLES AND TURMERIC RICE

When cells in the body are inflamed the body produces protein-like substances called kinins. Eating plenty of vegetables is known to reduce kinin production and activity, keeping inflammation under control. Another group of chemicals released by body cells during times of inflammation are called leukotrienes. Turmeric contains curcumin, which naturally inhibits the pro-inflammatory effects of these leukotrienes.

**Ingredients**

300g (10½oz) brown basmati rice
600ml (1 pint) vegetable
   or chicken stock
4 carrots
2 leeks
4 courgettes
2 onions

2 tablespoons olive oil
2 cloves of garlic
12mm (½in) fresh root ginger, grated
3 teaspoons turmeric
200g (7oz) cashew nuts
1 tablespoon chopped fresh coriander
Black pepper

**Method**

Rinse the rice and place in a saucepan with the stock. Bring to the boil, then turn down the heat and simmer for 30–40 minutes or until cooked. Drain and keep warm in the saucepan. Meanwhile, wash and chop the carrots, leeks and courgettes and place in a steamer. Steam for 15 minutes. Peel and chop the onions and garlic. Heat the oil in a large, deep frying pan. Add the onions and fry until they are transparent, then add the garlic, ginger and turmeric and cook for 1–2 minutes. Stir in the rice, steamed vegetables, cashew nuts and coriander. Heat through and season to taste with pepper. Garnish with a few coriander leaves.

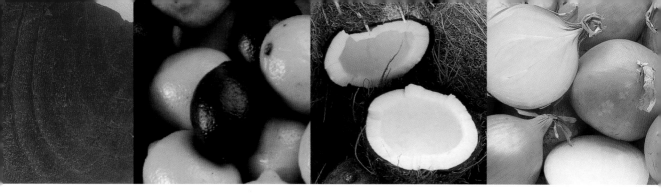

## SPICY TROPICAL FRUIT SALAD

Ongoing inflammation can result in tissue damage, fluid build-up and subsequent swelling. Pineapple contains the enzyme bromelain, which helps to dissipate fluid and swelling. Ginger contains natural anti-histamine, which blocks the body's production of pro-inflammatory hormones. This fruit combination can help to combat inappropriate inflammation.

**Ingredients**

2.5cm (1in) fresh ginger
175ml (6floz) water
4 star anise

1 pineapple
2 mangoes
2 papayas

**Method**

Peel and slice the ginger and place in a saucepan with the water and star anise. Bring to the boil and simmer for 3–4 minutes. Remove from the heat and leave to cool while you peel and chop the pineapple, mangoes and papayas. Place the fruit in a large bowl then, when it is cool, pour the ginger-infused liquid over the fruit. Serve with natural bio yoghurt or buckwheat pancakes.

## LEMON BALM AND GINGER ICED TEA

This tea can be drunk hot as a spicy tea in winter or cold as a refreshing drink over the summer months. Ginger has properties that have an antihistamine effect so if you suffer from ongoing pain and inflammation replace your daily cups of tea or coffee with this drink as part of your anti-inflammatory dietary plan.

**Ingredients**

5cm (2in) fresh ginger
1 large sprig of fresh lemon balm

1 litre (1¾ pints) boiling water

**Method**

Peel and slice the ginger. Wash the lemon balm. Pour the boiling water into a saucepan, add the ginger and lemon balm and cover with a lid. Leave to infuse for 10 minutes then either drink while hot or transfer to a large jug and chill until needed. It can be kept in the refrigerator for 2 days.

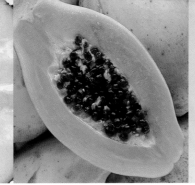
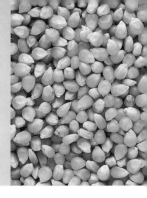

# Recipes for the heart and circulation

Dark red fruits and berries contain pro-anthocyanadins – compounds that are known to support the structure of the minute capillaries and larger blood vessels throughout the body. Oily fish contain the omega-3 group of essential fats that are thought to reduce the build-up of cholesterol plaques in the arteries and maintain general healthy heart function, while wholegrains provide the fibre needed to remove excess cholesterol from the digestive tract.

## THREE-SEED MUESLI

This recipe makes a large batch of muesli for you and your family to enjoy. The oat bran, a rich source of soluble fibre, is well renowned for reducing cholesterol levels and the seeds are rich in omega-6 essential fatty acids, which help to protect blood from becoming too sticky.

**Ingredients**

| | |
|---|---|
| 900g (2lb) porridge oats | 450g (1lb) oat bran |
| 250g (9oz) sunflower seeds | 200g (7oz) pumpkin seeds |
| 50g (2oz) sesame seeds | 200g (7oz) hazelnuts |
| 50g (2oz) coconut flakes | 250g (9oz) chopped dates |

**Method**   Place all the ingredients in a large bowl and mix together well. Store in a large air-tight container until needed. Serve for breakfast with rice, soya or cow's milk and a chopped banana or a tablespoon of natural yoghurt.

## VANILLA SMOOTHIE

If eating muesli every morning to keep your cholesterol low has become a little repetitive here is a great breakfast alternative. Bananas are rich in potassium, an important mineral for promoting healthy blood pressure.

**Ingredients**

| | |
|---|---|
| 4 bananas | 2 tablespoons oat bran |
| 1 litre (1¾ pints) rice or soya milk | 6 ice cubes |
| 3 teaspoons vanilla extract | |

**Method**   Place all the ingredients in a blender and blend until smooth. Pour into four glasses and serve straight away.

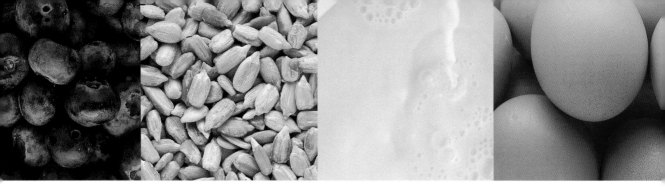

## TAHINI SALAD DRESSING

Your heart pumps blood at a consistent rate and pressure so that oxygen can be delivered to every cell in your body, from the tips of your toes to the top of your head. These cardiac rhythmic muscular contractions are regulated by two minerals – calcium and magnesium. Sesame seeds are rich in both, making this a hearty salad dressing.

**Ingredients**

5 tablespoons olive oil

1 tablespoon lemon juice

1 tablespoon white wine vinegar

2 tablespoons light tahini

**Method**

Place all the ingredients in a screw-top jar and shake well until a smooth consistency is reached. Drizzle over salad. It will keep for 1–2 weeks if refrigerated.

## THREE-BEAN SALAD

Ample daily dietary fibre is vital for efficient elimination of cholesterol, and beans and pulses (legumes) are one of nature's best sources of soluble fibre. This salad is packed full of fibre. Its natural sweetness from sweetcorn and peppers along with the summer basil flavour make it a great accompaniment to any protein dish.

**Ingredients**

240g (8½oz)black-eye beans

240g (8½oz) chickpeas

240g (8½oz) kidney beans

260g (9oz) sweetcorn

3 sticks of celery

1 red pepper

1 tablespoon roughly torn
  basil leaves

2 tablespoons flax or olive oil

Juice of 1 lemon

Black pepper

**Method**

Rinse and drain the black-eye beans, chickpeas, kidney beans and sweetcorn and place in a large salad bowl. Wash and finely slice the celery, then add to the salad bowl. Wash, de-seed and finely chop the red pepper and add to the salad bowl along with the basil. Drizzle on the flax or olive oil and the lemon juice. Thoroughly mix all the ingredients. Season to taste with pepper.

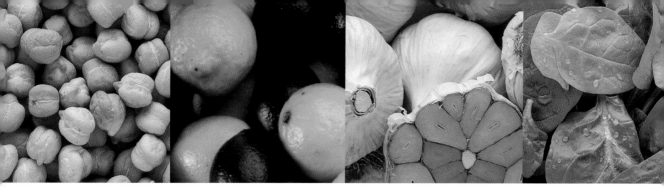

## HEALTHY HEART HOUMOUS

Red peppers and tomatoes are rich in bioflavanols, which can both protect blood vessel walls from damage and prevent blood fats from becoming oxidized and sticky. Cayenne pepper is a circulatory tonic and if you like hot food, then feel free to add ½ teaspoon to the ingredients.

**Ingredients**

2 large red peppers
175ml (6floz) light tahini
2 tablespoons flax or olive oil
1 tablespoon chopped fresh parsley
1 clove of garlic

6 sun-dried tomatoes
240g (8½oz) chickpeas
Pinch of cayenne pepper
Juice of 1–2 lemons

**Method**

Preheat the oven to 220°C/425°F/Gas 7. Place the red peppers on a baking tray and bake in the oven for 10 minutes or until cooked. Leave to cool, then peel, chop and de-seed the peppers. Place all the ingredients except for the lemon juice in a blender and blend on a high speed until smooth. Add the juice of 1 lemon, taste, and add more lemon juice if required. Place the houmous in a bowl and sprinkle with cayenne pepper before serving.

## SALMON WITH ROCKET AND PINE NUTS

This dish is packed with essential fats – salmon is rich in omega-3 fatty acids, and pine nuts in omega-6 essential fatty acids. Together these two families of oil help to protect the cardiovascular system and are also vital for brain function, the nervous system and healthy hair, skin and nails.

**Ingredients**

4 organic or wild salmon fillets
4 shallots
1 clove of garlic
1 tablespoon chopped fresh dill

1 tablespoon olive oil
15–20 rocket leaves per plate
100g (3½oz) pine nuts

**Method**

Preheat the grill. Rinse the salmon and place on a shallow baking tray. Peel and chop the shallots and garlic. Sprinkle the shallots, garlic, dill and olive oil over the salmon. Place the fish under the grill for 6–10 minutes, turn, and cook for a further 5–10 minutes or until cooked. Meanwhile, wash, dry and divide the rocket between four plates. Place the salmon next to the rocket and sprinkle with the pine nuts. Excellent served with fresh vegetables and a drizzle of cranberry dressing (see page 154).

Evening Meals

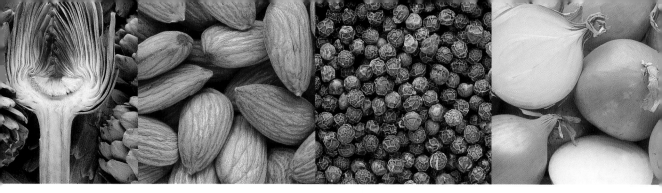

## HEARTY ROASTED VEGETABLES AND GARLIC

Peppers are rich in beta-carotene and other antioxidants that help to protect blood fats. Garlic has a strong traditional reputation for keeping the heart healthy and reducing blood cholesterol (roasting the garlic whole in its skin allows it to become sweet and soft). Once cooked, squeeze the garlic out of its skin and spread over the cooked vegetables.

**Ingredients**

3 red onions
3 yellow peppers
3 red peppers
3 orange peppers
1 aubergine
2 courgettes
10 cloves of garlic, unpeeled

4 tablespoons olive oil
1 tablespoon chopped fresh thyme
1 tablespoon chopped fresh rosemary
1 tablespoon chopped fresh oregano
1 tablespoon chopped fresh marjoram
Pinch of black pepper

**Method**

Preheat the oven to 180°C/350°F/Gas 4. Peel and quarter the onions. Wash, de-seed and quarter the peppers. Wash and chop the aubergine and courgettes into good-size chunks. Spread all the prepared vegetables and the whole garlic cloves (with their skins) over a large shallow baking tray. Sprinkle over the olive oil, herbs and pepper. Bake in the oven for 40–50 minutes or until well cooked and charred but not burnt on top. Eat with salad leaves or fish or chicken dishes.

## APRICOT AND SESAME FLAPJACKS

These really are a sweet treat since they contain butter and sugar in the form of honey. Whilst sugar isn't usually on The Food Doctor menu, these flapjacks are an occasional treat. The oats and apricots combine to give good fibre content and the ginger acts as a circulatory tonic.

**Ingredients**

300g (10½oz) butter or
     non-hydrogenated vegetable oil
200g (7oz) organic set honey
450g (1lb) porridge oats

1 tablespoon sesame seeds
1 tablespoon chopped dried apricots
½ teaspoon ground ginger

**Method**

Preheat the oven to 180°C/350°F/Gas 4. Grease a shallow baking tray. Melt the butter or heat the oil in a saucepan on a low heat, add the honey and stir until dissolved. Add all the other ingredients, mix thoroughly then pour into the baking tray. Bake in the oven for 25–30 minutes or until golden brown. Cut the flapjacks whilst still hot, but leave them in the baking tray until cooled.

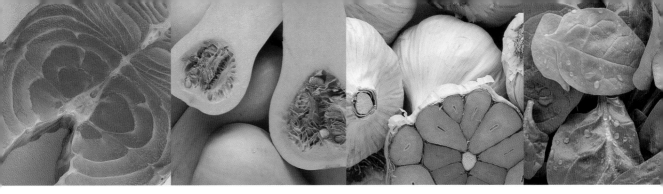

# Recipes to help protect against cancer

It is now accepted that food may play a part in the prevention and development of some cancers. Phyto-oestrogens, found in soya, seeds and other vegetables, may help regulate oestrogen dominance, one of the contributing factors in hormone-related cancers. Antioxidant nutrients, found in all red, yellow and orange fruits and vegetables, seafood, wholegrains and seeds, can quench exessive free-radical production, known to be associated with the development of many cancers. It is not claimed that foods can cure cancer, but it is thought that eating five to seven helpings of fresh fruit and vegetables daily reduces the incidence per capita of cancer.

## RAW CARROT, BEETROOT AND APPLE JUICE

There are many potential benefits of raw juicing for boosting immunity and perhaps increasing your protection from cancer. Although proper vegetable juice extractors are expensive, they are worth their weight in gold. Juicing takes no time at all and delivers a rapidly absorbable source of concentrated vitamins, minerals, antioxidants and health-boosting phytonutrients. This particular combination is one of our favourites because it is packed full of beta-carotene, pectin, vitamin C and bioflavanols and thus helps restore health and vitality.

**Ingredients**
6 large carrots
4 cooking apples
3 beetroot
Ice cubes

**Method**
Wash all the fruit and vegetables. Cut into suitable sizes for the juicer and juice. Serve chilled with ice cubes. It will keep in the refrigerator for up to 24 hours.

## MILLET AND FLAX OIL PORRIDGE

Keeping the body alkaline is of great importance when fighting cancer. Millet has an alkalizing effect on body tissues and is easy to digest – it can be used in the same way as porridge oats. Studies have shown that omega-3 oils found in flax seeds have anti-cancer properties, whilst pumpkin seeds are high in zinc, an immune-boosting mineral.

**Ingredients**
300ml (½ pint) water or rice milk
8 tablespoons millet flakes
1 teaspoon honey
1 tablespoon pumpkin seeds
2 tablespoons flax oil

**Method**
Pour the water or milk into a large saucepan and bring to the boil. Add the millet flakes and stir until it starts to bubble, then turn down the heat and simmer for 2–3 minutes. Add the honey and pumpkin seeds. Remove from the heat and leave for a couple of minutes. Add more rice milk or water if it is too thick. Stir in the flax oil, pour into bowls and serve with a chopped banana and sprinkling of cinnamon.

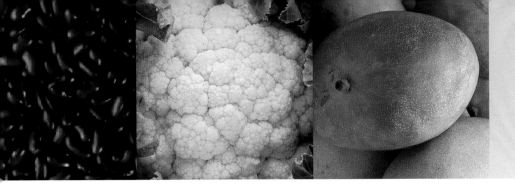

## SUMMER BERRIES AND SOYA YOGHURT

Soya yoghurt is rich in phyto-oestrogens, which protect against hormone-related cancers. Flax oil is known to have an inhibitory effect on cancer cell growth. Purple summer berries such as blueberries, redcurrants, blackcurrants and blackberries are rich in pro-anthocyanadins, which boost immunity.

**Ingredients**
1 tablespoon bio soya yoghurt
1 teaspoon flax oil

2 tablespoons mixed summer berries

**Method**
To make one serving place the yoghurt in a bowl and stir in the flax oil. Top with summer berries and it is ready to serve. Repeat for the number of people at breakfast.

## MISO SOUP

Miso is a traditional Japanese food made from fermented soya beans. The fermentation process increases the potency of soya phyto-oestrogens, which have long been known to protect against oestrogen-related cancers. This is a simple dish to make, but full of immune-boosting properties.

**Ingredients**
6 spring onions
100g (3½oz) water chestnuts
2 carrots
2 cloves of garlic
2.5cm (1in) fresh ginger

240g (8½oz) black-eye beans
1 tablespoon olive oil
1¼ litres (2 pints) fresh vegetable stock
1–2 tablespoons miso paste (dark or light)

**Method**
Wash and slice the spring onions, water chestnuts and carrots. Peel and finely chop the garlic. Wash and grate the ginger. Rinse and drain the black-eye beans. In a large saucepan, heat the olive oil, add the onions, garlic, ginger, carrots and water chestnuts and gently cook for 5–10 minutes or until the carrots start to go soft. Add the stock, black-eye beans and miso paste. Stir until the miso paste dissolves and bring to the boil for 1–2 minutes. Turn down the heat and simmer for a further 5 minutes then serve.

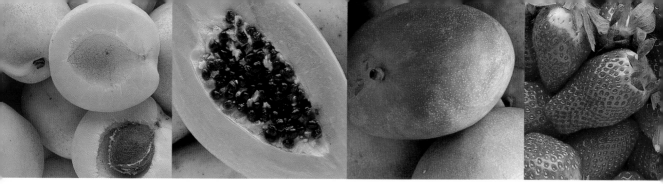

## ORANGE SPROUT SALAD

Oranges are high in vitamin C, a powerful antioxidant and anti-inflammatory agent. Sprouts are highly nutritious as they contain proteins, minerals, B vitamins and numerous types of antioxidants. Sprouted beans could be considered a perfect food as they are so nutrient dense, and growing your own is very easy and economical too – most health food shops now sell home sprouting kits.

**Ingredients**
1 orange
5 tablespoons alfalfa sprouts
3 tablespoons mung bean sprouts
2 tablespoons sunflower seeds
2 tablespoons flaked almonds
Oriental salad dressing (see recipe below)

**Method**  Peel the orange and slice into thin slithers. Wash and drain all the sprouts and mix them together in a large salad bowl, then add the orange. Sprinkle over the sunflower seeds and flaked almonds. Drizzle with Oriental salad dressing and serve.

## ORIENTAL DRESSING OR MARINADE

Tamari is traditional, naturally fermented soy sauce, full of immune stimulators and rich in flavour. Garlic helps to protect the body from infection whilst ginger is anti-inflammatory and adds a bit of bite to this delicious dressing.

**Ingredients**
1 clove of garlic
2 tablespoons tamari soy sauce
1 teaspoon grated fresh ginger
1 teaspoon honey
5 tablespoons sesame oil

**Method**  Peel the garlic and slice in half (or finely chop it if you are going to use this as a marinade). Place all the ingredients in a screw-top jar and shake until well mixed. Works well with any salad leaves. This will keep for 1–2 weeks in the refrigerator.

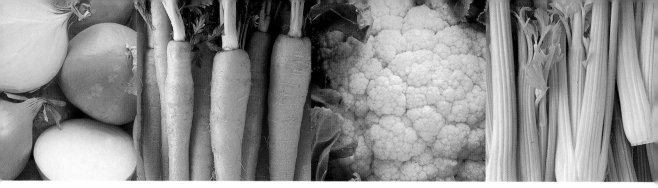

## PINTO BEAN AND BRAZIL NUT PÂTÉ

Selenium has a reputation for being a protective mineral against cancer. This mineral can help neutralize harmful chemicals, thereby slowing their activity. It is this free-radical quenching activity that makes selenium such an important immune protector, and Brazil nuts are a notable source of this vital mineral.

**Ingredients**

200g (7oz) Brazil nuts
1 large red onion
2 cloves of garlic
1 red chilli
1 tablespoon olive oil
Pinch of cayenne pepper

2 teaspoons mixed fresh or dried herbs
240g (8½oz) can of pinto beans
½ teaspoon paprika
1 tablespoon tomato purée
1 tablespoon lemon juice

**Method**

Grind the Brazil nuts to a powder. This is easiest if done in the coffee grinder attachment of a food processor. Peel and slice the onion and garlic. De-seed and finely chop the chilli. Heat the oil in a frying pan and fry the onions, garlic, chilli, cayenne pepper and mixed herbs together until soft. Place all the ingredients in a blender or food processor and blend on a high speed until a smooth consistency is reached. Add more water if the mixture becomes dry. Serve on rye toast, Ryvita, oatcakes or rice cakes. If you want to use it as a dip with crudités then thin with a little more water.

## WATERCRESS SOUP

Watercress is rich in vitamin C, which is a vital immune-boosting nutrient, as well as containing indoles, which help to generate a protective antioxidant enzyme.

**Ingredients**

1 large onion
2 medium leeks
1 tablespoon olive oil
4 large potatoes

2 bunches of watercress
600ml (1 pint) chicken or vegetable stock
Black pepper
¼ teaspoon grated nutmeg

**Method**

Peel and finely chop the onion and leeks. Heat the olive oil then add the onion and leeks and fry until soft. Wash and chop the potatoes into small cubes and add to the frying pan. Wash and chop the watercress and add to the pan. Add the stock, season with pepper and bring to the boil. Turn down the heat and simmer for 45 minutes. Remove from the heat and allow to cool slightly then pour the contents into a blender or food processor and blend until smooth. Return to the saucepan to reheat, then pour into bowls and serve with a sprinkling of nutmeg.

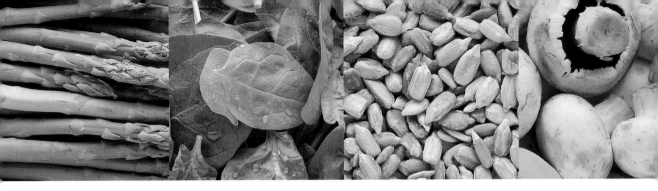

## MAGICAL MUSHROOMS AND SEA GREENS

These mushrooms have numerous immune- and anti-cancer properties. They are rich in beta-glucans, a powerful immune-stimulating nutrient, and are also high in protein. This dish is a great meal for anyone wanting to increase their protein intake without eating meat or fish.

**Ingredients**

400g (14oz) potatoes
100g (3½oz) shiitake, reishi or
  maitake mushrooms
300g (10½oz) button mushrooms
1 large brown onion
2 cloves of garlic

2 tablespoons olive oil
1 teaspoon paprika
250ml (8floz) vegetable stock
200ml (7floz) natural yoghurt
Black pepper

**Method**

Wash, peel and chop the potatoes into small cubes. Parboil them for 10 minutes then drain. Wash and slice the mushrooms. Peel and chop the onion and garlic. Heat the oil in a heavy-based deep frying pan and add the onion, garlic, mushrooms and paprika. Fry until brown, stirring occasionally. Add the stock and potatoes, turn down the heat and simmer for 10 minutes or until the potatoes are cooked. Remove from the heat and stir in the yoghurt. Season to taste with pepper and serve with brown rice.

## TOFU AND BROCCOLI STEAM-FRY

Broccoli is rich in indols, a plant substance that helps the body to fight cancer. Tofu contains phyto-oestrogens, known to be protective against many hormone-receptive cancers. Parsley and spinach are rich in both vitamin C and magnesium, which are needed for optimum immunity.

**Ingredients**

250g (9oz) plain tofu
Oriental marinade (see page 168)
1 large head of broccoli
150g (5oz) spinach
8 spring onions
1 bulb of bok choi

400g (14oz) carrots
2 tablespoons sesame oil
2 cloves of garlic
250ml (8floz) vegetable stock
4 tablespoons chopped fresh parsley

**Method**

Finely slice the tofu and marinate for 2–3 hours in Oriental marinade, then discard the marinade. Wash and roughly chop the broccoli, spinach, spring onions and bok choi. Wash, peel and slice the carrots. Heat the oil in a wok. Add the onions, garlic and tofu and cook for 4–5 minutes. Add the stock and bring to the boil, then add all the vegetables and the parsley. Cover and turn down the heat, steaming the vegetables for 4–6 minutes. Serve with brown rice, buckwheat noodles or rice noodles.

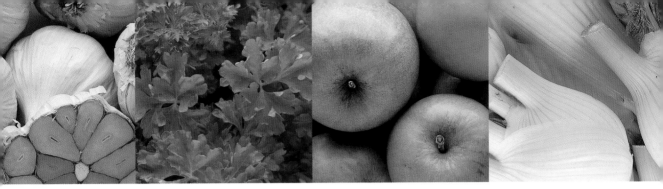

## SALMON AND MISO RISOTTO

Salmon is rich in omega-3 essential fats which help to fight cancer growth. Miso is rich in phyto-oestrogens, which help to protect against hormone-related cancers.

**Ingredients**
1 onion
1 clove of garlic
1 tablespoon olive oil
300g (10½oz) risotto rice
3 salmon fillets

750ml (1¼ pints) chicken or vegetable stock
2 teaspoons fresh miso
250g (9oz) green beans (with ends removed)
Juice of 1 lemon
Black pepper

**Method**
Peel and chop the onion and garlic. Heat the oil in a frying pan and add the onion and garlic and fry until soft. Add the rice and cook for a further 2–5 minutes. Add the salmon, stock, miso and green beans and cook for a further 20 minutes or until the rice is soft and all the stock has been absorbed. Add the lemon juice, season with pepper then serve.

## STEWED APPLE, PEAR AND FLAKED ALMONDS

Apples and pears are rich in pectin, a soluble fibre that helps to protect the health of normal body cells during or after radiotherapy. Almonds contain laetrile, a substance that helps to kill cancer cells.

**Ingredients**
2 large cooking apples
4 large pears
250ml (8floz) water
Juice of ½ lemon

½ teaspoon cinnamon
1–2 teaspoons honey
50g (2oz) flaked almonds

**Method**
Peel, core and chop the apples and pears and place in a heavy-based saucepan with the water, lemon juice and cinnamon and bring to the boil. Reduce the heat and simmer for 10–15 minutes or until the fruit has softened. Sweeten with honey to taste and serve sprinkled with flaked almonds. This dish makes a great accompaniment to home-made rice pudding (see page 151).

# glossary

**Absorption** The process by which nutrients are taken from the intestinal tract into the bloodstream, and into the cells in the body.

**Allergen** A substance (ingested or airborne) that promotes an allergic reaction.

**Amino acid** The breakdown product of protein. There are eight essential amino acids required by the body for rebuilding itself that must be derived from the diet, as the body cannot make them itself. See *Protein*.

**Anaemia** A condition that occurs when there are too few red blood cells in the body, or the haemoglobin levels are low (usually as a result of iron deficiency).

**Anaemia (pernicious)** Anaemia caused by vitamin B12 deficiency.

**Angina** Chronic chest pain and lack of ability to breathe caused by a narrowing of the arteries leading to the heart.

**Antacid** Over-the-counter medication to lower the acid levels in the stomach.

**Antibiotic** Medication that destroys bacterial infection.

**Antibody** Part of the immune system that neutralizes or engulfs invading pathogens.

**Antigen** An invader in the body that invokes an antibody reaction.

**Antihistamine** Medicinal or natural compound that prevents/suppresses the release of histamine.

**Antioxidant** A nutrient that slows the oxidative process caused by free-radical action.

**Arteries** Blood vessels that carry oxygen away from the heart to the rest of the body.

**Arteriosclerosis** The formation of plaque on the lining of an artery wall, caused by a build-up of cholesterol and other lipids and debris.

**Atherosclerosis** A thickening of the arterial walls, which impairs blood flow.

**Auto-immune disease** Occurs when the body starts reacting to its own tissue – examples are rheumatoid arthritis, multiple sclerosis, systemic lupus and diabetes.

**Bacteria** Microscopic germs. Some are friendly, others harmful.

**Benign** Non-cancerous cells.

**Beta-carotene** A precursor to vitamin A. A potent antioxidant.

**Bile** Secretion from the liver that helps break down fats in the digestive tract.

**Bioflavonoids** Compounds found just below the skin in fruits that aid the absorption of Vitamin C.

**Carcinogen** Any cancer-causing agent.

**Cardiac arrhythmia** Irregular heartbeat.

**Chemotherapy** A treatment for cancer using chemicals to kill the cancer cells.

**Cholesterol** A natural fat manufactured by the body to transport fatty acids, involved in hormone production.

**Co-enzyme** A molecule required by an enzyme to perform its work in the body. Required for the utilization of nutrients.

**Complex carbohydrate** Contains insoluble fibre within its structure that slows down digestion.

**Cruciferous** Family of vegetables known to possess anti-cancer properties, e.g. broccoli, cabbage and cauliflower.

**Detoxification** Process of getting rid of toxic matter from the body.

**Diuretic** Any substance that increases the rate of urination. A process of elimination and detoxification.

**DNA** Deoxyribonucleic acid – the genetic coding found in the nucleus of every cell in the body, which determines specific characteristics and function in the body.

**Endocrine** Glands in the body that release hormone for control of specific functions e.g. ovaries, testes.

**Endorphin** Natural substance produced in the brain that has painkilling properties.

**Enzymes** Molecules that break down proteins, involved in every reaction the body performs.

**Essential fatty acids** Substances that the body cannot manufacture by itself, but must be derived from the diet.

**Free radical** A single atom that is not paired with another, causing an imbalance in the electron chemical reactions in the body. They are produced as a natural waste product in the body, as part of an end product of metabolism, as well as being found in oils that have been overheated, or fried foods, etc. Very damaging.

**Fungus** Single-cell organisms that feed off a host, e.g. *Candida albicans* in the digestive tract.

**Gas** Excessive wind caused by bacterial or parasitic disturbance in the digestive tract.

**Gastritis** Inflammation of the stomach lining.

**Gastroenteritis** Inflammation of the stomach and intestines.

**Gastrointestinal** All parts of the digestive tract collectively.

**Genetic** Individual inherited characteristics.

**Gland** An organ that manufactures substances not required for its own metabolic activity.

**Haemoglobin** Part of the red blood cell that carries oxygen. Iron-dependent.

**Hair analysis** Non-invasive test whereby a small quantity of hair is removed from the nape of the neck for analysis of minerals and potential toxic substances.

**Hepatitis** Inflammation of the liver.

**Histamine** A chemical that is released from the body tissues that exerts a reaction in the smooth muscle tissues, e.g. constriction of the nasal and bronchial passages in hayfever or a wheal on the skin.

**Hormone** An essential substance produced by the endocrine glands that regulate body functions.

**Hydrochloric acid** Acid secreted in the stomach for the breakdown of proteins.

**Hyperallergenic** Being very susceptible to allergic reaction.

**Hypertension** High blood pressure.

**Hypoallergenic** Having little or no allergic reaction.

**Hypotension** Low blood pressure.

**Immune system** The body's collective force for protection against invading pathogens.

**Immunodeficiency** Having low immune function.

**Immunotherapy** Techniques used to stimulate the function of the immune system.

**Infection** Disease caused by invading bacteria, viruses or fungi.

**Insomnia** The inability to sleep.

**Insulin** Hormone produced by the pancreas to regulate glucose metabolism.

**Interferon** A protein produced by the immune system to fight viruses, and protect uninfected cells.

**Intestinal flora** Friendly bacteria found in the intestinal tract.

**Intrinsic flouactor** Compound produced in the stomach required for the absorption of vitamin B12.

**Leukaemia** Cancer that causes overproduction of white blood cells.

**Lipid** Fat or fatty substance.

**Lipoprotein** A protein bound to a lipid. Aids in the transport of fats around the arterial and lymphatic systems.

**Lymph** A clear fluid that flows around the lymph vessels, alongside the arterial system. Important for collecting debris and unwanted matter to be removed from the body, as well as carrying nourishment to the tissues.

**Lymph glands (or nodes)** Areas where the lymph collects viral, bacterial and waste products for filtering and engulfing by the immune system.

**Lymphocyte** A type of white blood cell which forms part of the immune system.

**Macrobiotic** A dietary approach eliminating all animal produce and being highly alkaline in its vegetarian content.

**Malabsorption** Lack of absorption of nutrients from intestinal tract to bloodstream.

**Malignant** Containing cancerous cells.

**Melanoma** A malignant growth originating from pigment cells in the skin.

**Menopause** A slowing of the production of hormones that regulate menstruation, and eventual ceasing of the menses.

**Metabolism** The production of energy brought about in the cells as a result of the breakdown of nutrients to glucose.

**Mucus membrane** The lining of any passage that has an opening to the outside of the body, e.g. ears, nose, mouth, anus and vagina.

**Naturopathy** Healing practice using herbs, tonics and body alignment for the rebalancing of the body to allow to it to heal itself.

**Neurotransmitter** A chemical that passes nerve impulses from one brain cell to another.

**Nutrients** Vital substances required by living beings for survival.

**Oncogenes** Cancer-promoting cells.

**Osteoporosis** Softening of the bones from deterioration of the bone tissue.

**Oxidation** A chemical reaction that results from exposure to oxygen. Can be potentially harmful.

**Parasite** An organism that lives off another organism or host.

**Pathogen** Any microorganism that causes disease, e.g. a parasite.

**Peroxides** Free radicals that result from the reaction between fats and oxygen.

**Phagocytosis** The engulfing of invading cells by immune cells to destroy them.

**Polyunsaturated fats** Fats that are derived from vegetables and seeds, e.g. flaxseed, sunflower and safflower oils. These oils should not be heated.

**Prostaglandin** A hormone-like substance that can promote or prevent inflammation.

**Protein** Complex compound formed from nitrogen which is essential to all living things. Required for growth and repair. Broken down into amino acids in the body.

**Quercetin** An anti-inflammatory compound.

**Saturated fats** Those fats that are derived from animal sources. Potentially damaging if overheated, and excessive amounts lead to arteriosclerosis and obesity.

**Serotonin** A neurotransmitter present in nerve cells, required for relaxation, sleep and concentration.

**Serum** The clear-coloured fraction of blood that carries the white and red blood cells.

**Simple carbohydrate** Processed foods that yield simple sugars which are broken down rapidly into glucose.

**Syndrome** A group of symptoms that characterize specific disease.

**T-cell** An immune cell that is responsible for attacking invading pathogens.

**Thrush** Fungal infection caused by overgrowth of *Candida albicans*.

**Toxicity** A poisonous reaction in the body that results from an overload of toxins, and the body's inability to clear them efficiently.

**Villi** Minute finger-like projections found throughout the length of the digestive tract that absorb nutrients.

**Virus** A minuscule molecule that infects host cells. Can cause major illness. Not affected by antibiotics.

**Vitamins** Essential nutrients that the body cannot manufacture itself, which must be derived from the diet.

**Yeast** A single cell organism that may cause infection in any canal of the body that is open to the outside, e.g. mouth, vagina and ears.

# useful addresses

## UK Organizations

**British Diabetic Association**
10 Parkway
London NW1 7AA
tel. 020 7424 1000

**British Heart Foundation**
14 Fitzhardinge Street
London W1H 6DH
tel. 020 7935 0185

**British Nutrition Foundation**
52–54 High Holborn
London WC1V 6RQ
tel. 020 7404 6504

**British Society for Mercury Free Dentistry**
P.O. Box 42606
London SW5 OXA
tel. 020 7373 3655

**Coeliac Society**
P.O. Box 220
High Wycombe
Buckinghamshire HP11 2HY
tel. 01494 437 278

**The Coronary Prevention Group**
2 Taviton Street
London WC1H OBT
tel. 020 7927 2125

**Eating Disorders Association**
First Floor, Wensum House
103 Prince of Wales Road
Norwich NR1 1DW
tel. 01603 621 414

**Foresight: the Association for the Promotion of Pre-Conceptual Care**
28 The Paddock
Godalming, Surrey GU7 1XD
tel. 01483 427 839

**The Institute for Optimum Nutrition**
13 Blades Court, Deodar Road
London SW15 2NU
tel. 020 8877 9993

**National Asthma Campaign**
Providence House
Providence Place
London N1 ONT
tel. 020 7226 2260

**National Eczema Society**
163 Eversholt Street
London NW1 1BU
tel. 0870 241 3604

**Society for the Promotion of Nutritional Therapy**
BCM Box SPNT
London WC1N 3XX

**The Soil Association**
Bristol House
40–56 Victoria Street
Bristol BS1 6BY
tel. 0117 929 0661

**Vegetarian Society of the United Kingdom**
Parkdale
Dunham Road
Altrincham
Cheshire WA14 4QG
tel. 0161 928 0793

**World Cancer Research Fund**
19 Harley Street
London W1G 9QJ
tel. 020 7343 4200

## US Organizations

**American Association for World Health**
1825 K St, N.W., Suite 1208
Washington DC 20006

**National Institute of Nutritional Education**
1010 S. Joliet Street 107
Aurora, CO 80012
800-530-8079

**American Cancer Society**
1599 Clifton Road North East
Atlanta, GA 30329
800-ACS-2345

**American Heart Association**
7272 Greenville Avenue
Dallas, TX 75231-4596
214-373-6300

**American Diabetes Association**
1701 North Beauregard Street
Alexandria, VA 22311
www.diabetes.org

**Crohn's and Colitis Foundation of America**
386 Park Avenue South, 17th Fl.
New York, NY 10016
800-932-2423

**Food Allergy Network**
11781 Lee Jackson Highway,
Suite 160, Fairfax VA 22033
800-929-4040

**Lupus Foundation of America**
2000 L Street, N.W., Suite 710
Washington DC 20036
202-349-1156

**Multiple Sclerosis Foundation**
6350 North Andrews Avenue
Fort Lauderdale, FL 33309
800-441-7055

**American Celiac Society**
P.O. Box 23455
New Orleans, Louisiana 70183-0455
504-737-3293

## Web Addresses

**Austin Nutritional Research**
www.realtime.net/anr/

**Center for Nutritional Research**
www.bovinecolostrum.com

**Food Science Central**
www.foodsciencecentral.com

**Harvard Medical**
www.harvardmed.com

**Tufts University Nutrition Navigator**
www.navigator.tufts.edu

# index

# acknowledgments

Jacket photography: Chrysalis Images/Nicki Dowey, except for centre photograph on front, Chrysalis Images/Neil Mersh and Jo Henderson

All other photography: Chrysalis Images/Neil Mersh and Jo Henderson, except for the following:

Chrysalis Images/Nicki Dowey: 1, 2, 3, 41 (top left), 43 (centre left), 43 (bottom right)

Chrysalis Images/Sian Irvine: 41 (bottom left)

Chrysalis Images/David Johnson: 45

Chrysalis Images/Michael Wicks: 22 (3rd from bottom), 41 (centre left), 43 (top left), 43 (centre right), 157 (top left)

Digital Vision: 38, 44

fabfoodpix.com: 46

Stockbyte: 40, 41 (bottom right), 42, 43 (bottom left)